Rebound 1980

LAUGHTER AND HEALTH

LAUGHTER AND HEALTH

BY

AMES J. WALSH, M.D., Ph.D., Sc.D., Litt.D., K.C.St.G.

MEDICAL DIRECTOR OF FORDHAM UNIVERSITY SCHOOL OF SOCIOLOGY;
PROFESSOR OF PHYSIOLOGICAL PSYCHOLOGY,
CATHEDRAL COLLEGE, NEW YORK

D. APPLETON AND COMPANY
NEW YORK :: 1928 :: LONDON

TO

Dr. John A. Foote

IN MEMORY OF THE OLD HOME TOWN,
ARCHBALD, PENNSYLVANIA, A SLIGHT
TOKEN OF APPRECIATION

PREFACE

This is a serious book on laughter. Laughter which is peculiar to man and is shared by none of the animals is a process very difficult to understand from its mental aspect, for no one has ever been able to explain satisfactorily just why our diaphragm goes into a series of convulsive movements whenever we hear or see anything funny. Indeed it is about as difficult to define what we mean by funny as what we mean by color. Try to think what you would say to a color-blind man to have him understand what you mean by red and then you will be able to appreciate how almost impossible it is to explain to a man without a sense of humor what you mean by "funny."

While laughter is a mystery from its mental aspect, it is easy to appreciate its far-reaching physical effects. The diaphragm, the principal organ involved in it, is in intimate anatomical relations with all the organs in the body that carry on the physical life. Whenever there are convulsive movements in the diaphragm, they are sure to be affected by them. As laughter always makes us feel better for having indulged in it, it is evident that the effect of the movements of the diaphragm and the large organs in its neighborhood is beneficial.

So far this favorable influence of laughter for the most important organs of the body has not been studied from the standpoint of therapeutics, that is, with the definite purpose of indicating how valuable it may be not only in conserving health but also in restoring it, if function alone has been disturbed and no organic changes have taken place. This is as far as medical therapeutics can go at any time. This volume is written to cover this field and indicate the good effects for health which flow directly from laughter and its favorable influence upon body and mind. There seems no doubt that hearty laughter stimulates practically all the large organs, and by making them do their work better through the increase of circulation that follows the vibratory massage which accompanies it, heightens resistive vitality against disease. Besides, the mental effect brushes away the dreads and fears which constitute the basis of so many diseases or complaints and lifts men out of the slough of despond into which they are so likely to fall when they take themselves overseriously.

The book gives the reasons why the cultivation of a habit of laughter is a potent factor for health, since through it an immense amount of organic stimulation can be secured in the most natural way without any risk of injury. The use of stimulants is the hardest thing in medicine to regulate properly but nature's own control safeguards laughter and prevents abuse.

J. J. W.

CONTENTS

A philosophical expert has enunciated the maxim: Civilization varies as the amount of soap used—$C \propto S$. In these days, however, of standardized production, of patent packages, scientific salesmanship and universal hygiene, soap has lost its diagnostic powers as a test of civilization. Soap is cosmopolitan. The maxim should be amended. After all, soap has no depth; it remains on the surface. A profounder and better measure of civilization is humor—$C \propto H$.

REV. FRANCIS P. DONNELLY, S.J., in *Literary Art and Modern Education*.

One excellent test of the civilization of a country I take to be the flourishing of the Comic idea and Comedy.

MEREDITH in *Essay on Comedy*.

The best formula for the health of the individual is contained in the mathematical expression: health varies as the amount of laughter—$H \propto L$.

LAUGHTER AND HEALTH

CHAPTER I

INTRODUCTION

LAUGHTER, according to the *Century Dictionary* is "a mode of expressing mirth, consisting chiefly in certain convulsive and partly involuntary actions of the muscles of respiration, by means of which, after an inspiration, the expulsion of the air from the chest in a series of jerks produces a succession of short abrupt sounds accompanied by certain movements of the muscles of the face and often of other parts of the body." The principal physical agent in laughter is the diaphragm or midriff as it is called in old-fashioned English, the large muscle which separates the abdominal region from the chest. This large muscle moves up and down in respiration over a distance of two or three inches according to the depth of the inspiration. In laughter it probably moves up and down from four to six inches and the jerky movements of it have considerable effect upon the im-

1

portant organs which have anatomical relations
with the diaphragm, to use scientific terminology,
or which in simpler language are lifted and lowered by the diaphragm in its movements. The
diaphragm may be so strenuously moved in laughing that we "get a stitch in our sides" from the
process, that is, one or more of the constituent
muscle bundles of the diaphragm go into a sort
of spasm.

As the heart and lungs lie just above the diaphragm and the liver and stomach and pancreas and spleen lie just below it, and as the
kidneys and the large and small intestines are all
affected by these movements of the diaphragm, it
is easy to understand that laughter must play a
rather important rôle in the life and health of
humanity. All of these important organs which
constitute the basis of our vegetative or physical life
are massaged, or at least pressed upon in such a
way as to modify their circulation of blood to a
marked extent. As the activity of these organs
very largely depends on the circulation which
reaches them, and as their functions must be influenced to a marked degree by the circulation
through them, it becomes easy to understand that

laughter must have a rather important place in the health of humanity.

This has been recognized in a sort of general way but not so as to make the specific beneficial action of laughter on health as clear as should be. We all know the old phrase, "laugh and grow fat," and there is no doubt at all that people who laugh easily and heartily are much more likely to be healthy, and to continue in good health, than those who are almost never heard to laugh out loud, and whose highest attempt at mirth is likely to be a very quiet smile.

Laughing is distinctive of man. No animal laughs. Some of them make noises resembling laughter and these noises are sometimes spoken of as laughter but the word is used equivocally. Darwin, in his book on the expression of the emotions, suggested that "laughter seems primarily to be the expression of mere joy or happiness." No one would associate either of these words, however, with the animals who are sometimes said to laugh. The prowling animals, the jackal and the hyena, are described as laughing, but no one who knows anything about the habits of the animals in question would say that the sounds which they make, and which happen accidentally to be reminiscent of laughter, represent in any sense of the word what we call laughing in human beings.

It is true that certain of the domesticated animals, for instance the dog, often expresses pleasure in his countenance in something of the same way that pleasure is expressed by human beings when they smile, but there is all the difference in the world between this smiling and the associated movements of the diaphragm which are called laughter.* Note was taken of this fact that no animal laughs by the philosophers of the very old time, and it was the custom among them to declare that it is just as good a definition of man to say that he is "a risible animal" as to say that he is a rational animal. Man is the only animal that

---

* There is what is termed canine laughter in human beings, which is a facial expression resulting from spasm of the canine muscle, as it is called, or, in anatomy, *levator anguli oris* (the elevator muscle of the corner of the mouth). When this muscle is brought into action to an extreme degree, as it is by strychnine poisoning, the corners of the mouth are drawn up showing the side teeth as is done by a dog in snarling. This is also called the *risus sardonicus*, or sardonic smile. This latter adjective comes from the fact that a plant in Sardinia produces a similar effect to that of strychnine on these muscles. Any forced smile usually takes on this character. The fact that canine and sardonic laughter are synonymous shows how little mankind usually associates the idea of real laughter with the dog.

laughs. It is often thought in the modern time that the evolutionists brought us to the realization that man was an animal, but of course the philosophers for nearly three thousand years have been insisting on the animality of man with the rational quality attached. We have always been sure about the animal part of man, though not so sure about the rational. The risibility of mankind, however, has given him a distinction from the animal that is almost more differential than his rationality.

It has been suggested that laughter in physical terms is a reflex activity of the diaphragm, which moves up and down rapidly, drawing the air into the lungs in deep drafts, and expelling it forcibly, but interruptedly, through the larynx, with the production of certain elementary sounds, whenever we are tickled. The tickling may be either physical or mental. Physical tickling is represented by the sensations which are produced when we are subjected to a succession of touches in certain parts of the body. There are certain especially sensitive areas which, when touched lightly, bring as a reflex the up and down movement of the diaphragm which constitutes the principal activity in laughter. Tickling in children, if not violent, gives pleasure, though in older people there is usually an unpleasant sensation attached to it, a feeling of annoyance that may rise even to a definite sense of extreme discomfort, followed by lack of control of the nervous system.

Why touches of this kind in these special areas should produce laughter we do not know, any more than we know why the presence of dust, and especially certain irritating particles in the nose will bring about a sneeze, or why remaining in still air of equable temperature for some hours causes yawning. These two are diaphragm activities of a more or less convulsive kind and therefore related to laughter. Individuals differ very much in their reactions to such factors and there are certain mental elements that always enter into the cases. Children are very ticklish, but if a stranger should attempt to tickle them, instead of laughing they almost inevitably cry. Tickling the sole of the foot will always cause the foot to be rapidly withdrawn, but there will be no laughter unless there has been some anticipation of the touch. With some people, on the other hand, the reflex is excessive, with resultant lack of control of the nervous system, and even slight tickling may set up hysterical laughter that can scarcely be repressed.

There is as much individual difference as regards the response to mental tickling as there is to physical tickling. Certain incongruities of thought and unexpected relations and contrasts of thought and word cause us to have an intellectual reflex, as it were, that leads to laughter. Some people are ever so much more inclined to react to this mental tickling than others. We say that they have a good sense of humor. Some people actually have such a slight mental reflex in the direction of laughter, though often they are quite as intelligent as average people, that we say of them that they have no sense of humor. We pity them, but feel that they are not quite responsible for the deficiency and that it is part of their nature. On the other hand there are some people who are very much inclined to laugh and who laugh on the slightest occasion and find it rather difficult to control the reflex in this direction.

Age has much to do with both the physical and mental reflexes toward laughter. Children laugh rather readily, and begin to laugh from the very early months of life. In infants there seem to be many more gelasmogenic, or laugh-originating (to translate that Greek term into English), zones than in adults. Slight touches under the chin, or the rubbing of the scalp, or little touches anywhere in the abdomen, or along the anterior parts of the legs of infants will be followed by laughter almost as promptly as from touches along the ribs. On the other hand in old age the ticklish areas have almost entirely disappeared and touches over them are unpleasant rather than pleasant. The reaction is likely to be one of distinct annoyance.

Many books have been written about laughter and the cause of it, and many theories have been elaborated with regard to it, and yet no one thinks that we understand it in any adequate fashion. Just why certain incongruities of thought and similarities of words happen to make us laugh is very hard to understand. It is natural for man to laugh and yet there is no doubt that environment has much to do with it. If we have lived most of our lives under circumstances where we heard comparatively little laughter, we are likely to laugh very little. On the other hand, if we have been brought up in the midst of hearty laughing, we are almost sure to laugh heartily and easily. In a word laughter especially hearty laughter is as much dependent on habit as on nature.

There seems to be a certain distinction in the laughter of the two sexes, and women laugh much less readily and heartily than men as a rule, but this is attributed not so much to nature as to nurture. Women are—or used to be—brought up with the idea that they should repress more of their feelings than men, and the result is that they smile quietly or laugh very gently over jokes that cause their husbands or brothers to burst out into a gale of laughter. Whether in the new dispensation, when women feel less under the necessity of repressing themselves than before, there will be heartier laughter from the female of the species remains to be seen.

What we are interested in here is the fact that laughter from its physical make-up affects the large and most important organs of the body in such a way as to modify their function in the direction of the stimulation of it. As a result of that laughter has a distinct place in therapeutics, or at least in the realm of the maintenance of health. Manifestly laughter has a very definite purpose in life; or if the purpose of things should not appeal to one, then there seems to be no doubt that the human beings who laugh heartily and frequently, because they stimulate the large organs that lie along their diaphragm, have by that very fact a survival factor through which more of them live their lives out and leave offspring after them than do others. Hence all men laugh more or less, but those who laugh the most are the ones that live the longest and enjoy the best health.

It has often been said that it is not work but worry that shortens life, and the truth of this old saw is very generally accepted. The best way to get rid of worries is to laugh them off, for worry is getting into a disturbed state of mind over what you have to do next week, while you are trying to accomplish what you have to do to-day—though by next week what you were worrying about last week may prove to be a pleasure rather than a hardship, or may not have to be done at all.

It is a matter of common knowledge that the patients who suffer from the functional nervous troubles take themselves too seriously. Instead of hoping for the best they are always inclined to dread the worst. Sensations that are often scarcely more than physiological and that sometimes are actually natural are considered to be the symptoms of disease, and are supposed to represent at least threats of serious developments. The number of these nervous ailments has been increasing very much in recent years. The statistics of any such conclusion would be hard to find, but we have an abundance of evidence for it from the tremendous increase in the number of quacks and charlatans of all kinds who are making a very good living. We have all sorts of healers who are curing people. There are religious healers of all kinds. Nearly every important hotel in our larger cities has, during the winter time, somebody who hires one of the assembly rooms to preach some form of healing religion. Men, and particularly women, are cured by healing religions of the most absurd kind. There is "the religion of the solar plexus" which makes a good living for its high priest, and Dowie, who said that he was Elijah returned to earth, claimed to have touched and healed 200,000 people. There was no doubt at all that he "touched" them, and they themselves said they were healed, so that the religious idea proves very efficacious.

Dowie died under a cloud that made it very

clear that there could be nothing like any intimate contact between him and "the power that makes for righteousness in this world," and after that fiasco it would seem as though we would have no more such healers. Dowie was scarcely dead, however, before Schlatter turned up as a healing prophet in Denver. What surprised New Yorkers was that these self-proclaimed special messengers from the Deity should come to Chicago and Denver, unless perhaps on the principle that no places needed them so much. Schlatter, on the strength of his proclamation of his prophetship, proceeded to "cure" a lot of people, and they gathered in a line blocks long waiting to see him. He offered to send handkerchiefs blest by the prophet—perhaps containing some of his emanations—to those who could not come to Denver to see him, and for awhile, there was a very interesting correspondence school of healing. After a time, however, the United States postal authorities declared that handkerchiefs worth a few cents—they were not even linen—sent through the mails at ten dollars per, represented a fraud, and they issued a fraud order that banned Schlatterism for a while, but not before a great many people had been healed by Schlatter.

Nor did it prevent the continuance, for years, of his personal work as a healer.

It is easy to understand, then, that people are being cured of what they think serious ills by just being converted to not thinking too much about themselves, and not taking themselves too seriously. A distinguished French physician, who sees a great many neurotic cases, said that he thought that something more than half of all the nervous cases who come to see him have a persuasion of illness, a mental attitude that keeps up their symptoms rather than any physical ailment. To get them to change this attitude of mind is a very difficult matter, but sometimes the prophets succeed in doing it.

Any one who wants to read Dr. Still's own autobiography—he was the founder of osteopathy—will find that the old man believed that he had a special message from on high to cure people by his method. He used to say to his *diplomats*, that is to the graduates of his school, on whom he was conferring diplomas at their commencement, "Remember there is one God, one faith and one baptism, and one mode of healing all disease, osteopathy." It is this mystical element, much more than anything physical about it, that gave osteopathy its vogue at the beginning, though now of course there is the claim of marvelous physical therapeutics in connection with it.

The people who get cured by these quacks in our time are not the ignorant but the well-to-do and the more or less educated. Some of them are prominent merchants and lawyers and above all, they are the wives of the middle and upper classes, rather than the lower classes. One thing that education is doing for people is that it makes them more serious than they used to be. They learn to take themselves very seriously. There is not nearly so much hearty laughter as there used to be, or as there is even yet among country people, and especially the workers on the farms—the farmer himself is more stolid—and the laborers who are not affected by the city atmosphere. They are tempted to laugh and joke continuously at their work, but in the general population there is ever so much less hearty laughter than there used to be.

It has often been said that the reason for the increase in nervous symptoms in our time is that we are living the strenuous life, and men are deeply intent on a few things, and profoundly preoccupied. There is a great deal of truth in this, but the principal part of the truth is that men laugh ever so much less than they did before, and laughter is an extremely important element for health. This can be seen because of the extremely important organs just above and below the diaphragm, which it affects.

We have already said that women not only laugh ever so much less than men, but that they laugh ever so much less heartily. When they permit themselves a smile they do not as a rule go to the extent of laughing deeply. Some years ago that could be explained on the score that their corsets prevented them from having as free movement of their diaphragm as men can enjoy. The corset has gone, but the tendency for women not to laugh heartily remains, and undoubtedly this accounts for not a little of their tendency to suffer from functional nervous affections. They take themselves too seriously and do not permit themselves to enjoy the relaxation of hearty laughter.

In the sickness survey, that is the collection of morbidity statistics, made for a term of over two years by the United States Public Health authorities in the city of Hagerstown, Maryland, it was found that nervous affections, meaning thereby the non-organic nervous complaints, are more than three times as frequent among women as they are among men. Hagerstown is considered by the United States Health authorities to represent a cross section of American life, for it is not a large city, it is not particularly healthy, and may very well be taken as representative of the health and sickness of the United States generally, city and country.

It might be concluded that this greater tendency on the part of women to develop nervous symptoms is really due to the fact that they are more delicate of constitution, and therefore more likely to lose control of their nervous systems. In a word, it might seem to be natural and not acquired in any sense, the result of heredity as conjoined with sex, and not environment. During the Great War, however, we found that young men, when because of the war, they took themselves very seriously and did not laugh so much as they ought, suffered as much from nervous diseases as women might have been expected to. Indeed, the nurses who went out with the American Expeditionary Force suffered less from nervous affections—"shell shock" as the psychoneurotic affections were euphemistically called during the war—in proportion to their numbers than did the young men. Yet these nurses were often exposed to bursting shells and to the dangers of war as much as the men.

It would seem that there is something in the habits of the two sexes, that is, in their environment and its conditions, that has more to do with the difference between them as regards the development of nervous symptoms, than is to be found in their difference of nature. One of the most striking elements of this difference is to be found in the laughter of the two sexes, so that it is well worth while considering the influence that this may wield for health and for such relaxation of mind and body as may enable people to maintain control of themselves.

Something like laughter would seem to have been needed in order to replace for men that freedom of organic movement within the great cavities of the body, which is so striking in animals and so lacking in men. This is due to the difference of organic relaxation which occurs because the animal goes on all fours and man walks in the erect position. In the animal abdomen, for instance, all the large organs fastened to the backbone swing rather freely as the animal walks. Gravity tends to have them hang down against the abdominal muscles and they are supported by these, but are very much rubbed upon by the action of the muscles when the animal walks, particularly when the animal runs. The same thing is true, though not to so marked a degree, in the animal chest.

In man the conditions are quite different. All the organs are fastened to the backbone, but the erect position causes them by gravity to rest upon each other, to a certain extent at least, or upon the diaphragm. They do not swing as freely as in the abdomen and chest of the animals, where the back-bone is horizontal and everything hangs from it. When the animal moves rapidly there is a good deal of rubbing of the organs on one another. This is true also in man, but not to so great a degree. Of course, when he jumps the organs are set to flopping upon one another very much in the same way as in the rapidly moving animal. As man gets older, however, he stops jumping to a great extent, and even does away with all rapid movements, and so he needs something to replace the effect of these upon his organs in the erect position which he maintains.

When human beings sit down all their organs are

crowded together to a considerable extent, and there is very little movement of them, and it is not surprising that circulation in them should become sluggish. For if movements of organs on each other are necessary in order to stimulate the circulation, as seems to be very definitely true in both animals and men, then, just in proportion as we have become a sedentary people, we have lost the good effect of movement in bringing about organic friction and massage.

Laughter may be looked upon as an invention of nature to compensate for the diminution of organic friction and massage among the organs consequent upon man's erect position. Gravity tends to keep human organs much more at rest and with much less rubbing upon each other than is true of the animal. They are all in conditions of much greater stability than is true of the pendulous state in which they exist in animals. The sedentary habits of mankind, which are cultivated in association with civilization and its quieter ways, bring about the still greater suppression of organic movements. We need something like the jerky vibration which occurs in connection with the convulsive movements of the diaphragm during hearty laughter. All this has been known before, but the therapeutic quality of laughter has not been valued as it should be.

Some of the writers on humor of the older time have been convinced that laughter had a definite effect upon the health. Unfortunately, most of what Aristotle said with regard to laughter has been lost, though we know that he touched upon the subject, and even is said to have made a list of the various kinds of jokes. He thought of laughter as representing a sort of bodily exercise and he commended this kind of exercise as a precious function for the conservation of health. Some of the medieval authors of laughable stories, and especially those which represent a combination of prose and verse, talked of the health-giving qualities of laughter. The old French *fabliau* or *conte á rire en vers* was said to have a *vertu saine*, a sanitary, or health virtue. Indeed, it seems very likely that many of these old writers recognized the therapeutic qualities of laughter, but without our knowledge of the diaphragm and its relations, and what its up and down excursions might do in the massaging of all the important organs of the body, they were not in a position to point out just what was accomplished by good, hearty laughter. All they knew was that people felt better after it, that they digested better as the result of it, and that they slept better if they had spent the evening indulging in it.

We need laughter for the maintenance of health, and above all for that relaxation of mind and body which keeps us from taking ourselves too seriously. It has seemed, then, that attention ought to be called particularly to the value of laughter as a therapeutic agent. As will be seen in the course of the book, laughter affects deeply all the organs, but it also affects the mind in a very beneficial way. There is even a chapter on "Laughter and Surgery" which shows that during the War those who suffered very severely from shell wounds, and other serious injuries, got along ever so much better in hospitals where an air of cheeriness, with definite tendencies to the outbreak of laughter, at times prevailed, than in those in which an air of solemnity reigned. Men will die with a smile and a jest on their lips and be happy for it. After all that greatest of the English lord chancellors, the only man who cleared the docket of the court of chancery in England, a great intellectual genius, but a man of marvelous character and will power, who went to his death calmly for his opinions, Sir Thomas More, joked to the last. He said to the headsman, at the very foot of the scaffold, "Help me up these steps." (He was muscle bound after his long imprisonment.) "As for my coming down, you can let me shift for myself." As he was putting his head on the block, his beard, grown long in prison, got in the way so he pushed it aside, with the last words, "This has committed no treason."

Who would venture to say that this laughing tone is not a better way to face suffering, and even death, than the over conscious solicitude which adds to pain and makes it harder to bear. The Irishman said, "Life is a dangerous thing at best, and very few of us get out of it alive," but that constitutes all the more reason why we must take it as it comes. Laughter was manifestly given us to make life bearable even in the midst of the trials and suffering that are at some time or other practically inevitably associated with it. It has been said that in a life where there is death there is no room for hate, and it might be inferred that in a life where there is death, laughter becomes almost impossible, but that is only for the man who is a craven at heart, and who does not face things as they are. The laughter of men is the happiest sound we have, and its effect on the individual represents the most important relief that we possess for the trials mental and physical that are sure to find their way into life. I have known men living under what seemed almost impossible conditions who have found their refuge in life in laughter.

On last Bastille Day Paris indulged itself in the luxury of what it called "The Parade of the Massacred Faces." They were the five thousand living dead men of France, men who were wounded seriously in the face during the War. The conditions that have resulted in some cases are so hideous that even hospital surgeons accustomed to repair work turn away from them shocked at the sight. Some of the men had their faces completely torn away.

It is easy to understand the profound impression this procession produced along the boulevards in Paris, and yet practically all of these men know how to laugh, and they joke among themselves, and they find that there is still amusement in life. Those of them who have not been able to laugh have either died as the result of the depression that ensued, or have committed suicide. The New York *World* correspondent, writing about the effect produced on others by the sight of this awful procession, said that "strong men gnashed their teeth and women went into hysterics. There was a silence that froze the usually colorful boulevard into horror." It is easy to understand that something like this would take place, and yet it was not for the sake of the pity that they would arouse that the men marched, but because they felt that it was well for the world to know that this was the harvest of war, and at the same time to appreciate that men can live down even a supreme misfortune of this kind and laugh in the face of fate, even though there should not be much or almost no face to laugh with. They thus gave effective demonstration that men can be brave in peace as well as in war.

CHAPTER II

LAUGHTER AND THE LUNGS

U NDOUBTEDLY the most important effect of laughter on the human tissues is produced upon the lungs. When the diaphragm goes up and down in the course of laughing, large drafts of air are drawn into the lungs and then are forcibly ejected, causing the well-known sounds in the larynx, only to make room for more and more air until every portion of the lungs is thoroughly ventilated. The expansion of the chest by the lifting up of the ribs by means of the accessory muscles of respiration, which act very vigorously when the laughing is hearty, together with the downward movement of the diaphragm, increases the air content of the thorax by probably one half, and surely more than one third more than normal. As the result of this large quantities of air find their way into the lungs, only to be driven out again and again as the laughter proceeds.

By placing a thin person in the proper light and watching the sides of the chest closely, the diaphragm, as pointed out by Litten, some twenty-five years ago, can be seen as a sort of shadow to detach itself from the internal chest wall and move downward in deep breathing. Its excursions along the chest wall are two and one-half to three inches, and probably sometimes even more. Laughter encourages these excursions to the fullest extent, and this exercise of the lung function oxidizes the blood very thoroughly.

This thoracic expansion in deep inspiration draws an abundance of oxygen into intimate relation with the lung capillaries in the alveoli, or terminal chambers of the bronchioles, and oxygen is the most vitalizing material that we have. With it life may be prolonged when otherwise death would inevitably take place, though of course, if nature has not definite recuperative power, oxygen is only of temporary value. It used to be the custom to recommend deep breathing for those who were at all delicate in health, provided of course their delicacy of health did not come from pulmonary tuberculosis. When that disease is present, rest is the most important therapeutic agent for the lungs, and the exercise of pulmonary tissues required for deep breathing might readily endanger the tearing of capillaries, or the rupture of minute arterioles, with consequent hemorrhage. The practice of recommending deep breathing is still encouraged by hygienists, though to nothing like the same degree that used to be the custom. We prefer now to have people live in good fresh air, and sleep with their windows open, and therefore always be in the midst of an abundance of air that has not been contaminated by the breathing of other people, rather than have recourse to artificial aëration by conscious deep breathing.

It may be said at once, however, that it is well recognized that even the deepest voluntary breathing that we can exercise will not approach in thoroughness the effect of good breezy laughter. Most people need to have their tissues highly vitalized by the presence of liberal amounts of oxygen, and yet if they follow sedentary occupations, and are inclined to be sedate and tranquil in their movements, there is very little opportunity for them to secure that amount of oxygen which they ought to have in order to be thoroughly stimulated by its presence in the tissues everywhere throughout the body.

Gusts of laughter, as they are so aptly called, set

every portion of the lungs in movement because of the far-reaching expansion and contraction of the chest, and this brings about the ventilation of many back eddies of air space within the lungs which, under ordinary conditions, obtain renewal of their fresh air only by the slow process of the diffusion of gases. Certain portions of the lungs in a great many quiet people are very much less active than they ought to be because their possessors never breathe deeply. One of the best results of exercise, not merely quiet walking, but active rapid movements, is that it causes deep rapid breathing, and this brings about a thoroughgoing change of air in the lungs and a complete vitalization of the blood, that will immediately afterwards be distributed throughout the tissues.

It might very well seem that the very brief time, comparatively speaking, during which laughter lasts would preclude the possibility of laughter having very much effect on the oxidation of the blood, even though the lungs and diaphragm are the principal agents in laughter. Once it is realized, however, how rapidly the blood circulates, the effect of even brief intervals of laughter will be better understood. The blood represents somewhere between 5 and 7 per cent of the body weight, and nearly one-fourth of it at any one time is in the heart and lungs and large blood vessels. All the blood in the body passes through the lungs in the ordinary course of circulation oftener than once a minute. Even though a laugh should last not longer than a minute then all the blood in the body would have been exposed to the action of two or three times as much oxygen as when breathing was quiet and ordinary. Laughing for two or three minutes exposes the blood to three or four times as much oxidation at least as does quiet respiration, so that there is no wonder that a good hearty laugh makes us tingle with renewed vitality out to the very ends of our fingers and toes. In the course of a single minute every cell of tissue in the body, including the brain cells, will have been exposed to an increased amount of oxygen as a consequence of a hearty laugh.

Ordinarily we think of the circulation of the blood in the body as being a methodical round of rather sluggish flow. Any one however who has seen the blood in the veins of a frog's foot rushing along, the corpuscles jostling each other as the current hurries through the capillaries, is not likely to think of blood circulation as sluggish. Other experimental observations, however, have made the rapidity of the circulation of the blood very clear. For instance, if certain delicate re-agents are introduced into the jugular vein on one side of an animal's head, their presence may be detected in the jugular on the other side in much less than a minute, demonstrating that in the mean-time, this blood has gone back to the right heart, been sent on to the lungs for oxidation, returned from there to the left heart, and been sent out to the general circulation, and now is returning through a vein once more to begin its faithful round of the body again. That picture is likely to make one feel that anything which, like laughter, affects the lungs deeply is sure to produce a very definite and almost immediate effect, not only upon the blood, but through that, on all the various portions of the body. Not only do the muscles and the capillary circulation of the surface get this in-creased oxidation, but also the large organs, so that all of them are stimulated to do their work better. No wonder then that laughing after meals means so much for digestion and good feeling. Of course, exercise has the added advantage of stimulating, that is, making a special call on the heart, as the result of which that precious muscle pump sets the blood flowing faster and at a higher pressure, but the added oxidation of the lungs is an extremely valuable accessory without which, almost needless to say, the more rapid action of the heart would be utterly ineffective in enabling the muscles to keep up their active work.

A great many people as they get older, however, seldom get any exercise except that of quiet walking, which only very rarely causes the heart to beat faster and the lungs to make deeper excursions. They need something to stir up their functions and vitalize their systems, and nothing probably is better for this than laughter. Its effect upon the lungs is easy to understand, and the deep breathing that it inevitably leads to represents a very potent factor in stimulating not only the lungs, but practically all the organs of the body. Nature has made it extremely easy for young folks to laugh. Very little occasion is needed. By a sort of instinct they find even the slightest incongruities so amusing that they laugh heartily over them. As we grow older it is harder to make us laugh heartily, and some people seem to think that it is almost incompatible with the dignity of middle life and beyond to permit themselves to laugh cordially and deeply. Fortunately, while nature gradually takes away from us the power to exercise strenuously, or at least makes it a little dangerous to indulge in it, she leave us the precious faculty of laughter, and there are ever so many good reasons why we should allow ourselves to be tempted to make liberal use of it. It is the man who keeps up his activities as the years advance, as a rule, who lives longer than others, and the men and women who keep up their youthful habits with regard to hearty laughter who enjoy better health than the rest of mankind. Laughter is usually looked upon as an effect of good health, but it must not be forgotten that it is also a cause, and that there is a virtuous circle of influences formed between laughter and health.

How salutary for health the thoroughgoing change of air in the lungs, such as occurs during hearty laughter, may be, is very well illustrated by the current theory with regard to the initial lesion of pulmonary tuberculosis. There is a very prevalent impression among those who have had most experience with tuberculosis that the disease secures a foothold in the lungs, particularly in those portions where the air does not move so actively as in other parts. The apexes of the lungs, and especially the right apex, are particularly likely to be the site of tuberculous lesions, and, indeed, are considered to be the favorite point of attack of the disease. The reason for this peculiarity of the disease is usually that the air in contact with the tissues of the apex is not actively changing, because there is, as it were, an eddy in the lung ventilation in this area. The lack of full vitalization of the pulmonary tissues by oxygen makes them less resistive to the invasion of disease, hence the frequency with which tuberculosis occurs at these points.

The other portions of the lungs which are most frequently attacked are the margins, and here, too, there is less likely to be thorough ventilation than in the median parts of the lungs. Tuberculosis implantation and progress are said to be favored by sluggishness of ventilation of certain parts of the lungs.

Whenever there is much laughter these eddies of more or less stagnant air are thoroughly flushed out and fresh air finds its way to the very ends of the alveoli, and is likely to be changed thoroughly a number of times if the laughter continues for any length of time. Under these circumstances the resistive vitality of the lungs is greatly heightened and the chance of the implantation of the bacillus of tuberculosis, or indeed of any other microörganism very much lessened.

It has been pointed out that especially in the lungs this question of vital resistance is more important than elsewhere. The ordinary feeling is that if a bacterium finds its way into our respiratory tract it will produce the specific disease with which it is associated. This is not true, however, of the bacteria which produce respiratory disease. The germ of pneumonia, for instance, and also of certain of the bronchitises are to be found in our mouths and other parts of the upper respiratory tract rather frequently, even when we are in good health. If we have good resistive vitality, they may stay there for a prolonged period without producing symptoms of the disease. In a word the personal resistive vitality of the patient is more important than the virulence of the microbe. The resistive vitality is heightened by deep breathing and thoroughgoing oxidation of the tissues, and as this is greatly favored by laughter, indeed probably better than by any other mode of exercise, it is easy to understand that laughter of itself may be an extremely valuable agent, and probably often is the best adjuvant for the prevention of the development of respiratory disease.

Quite apart from what is accomplished in the lungs themselves, however, the amount of air which finds its way into the respiratory tract during laughter acts directly through the blood in bringing about stimulation of all the tissues in the body. No wonder that a good hearty laugh is such a stimulant for the circulation that we can feel the effects of it out to the very ends of our extremities.

There is certainly no drug that we have, and no stimulant that men are accustomed to, that produces so immediately anything like the same effect as a hearty laugh in setting all the tissues on edge for whatever action may be called for. Even in war, at the zero hour, it was noticed that the men who were readiest to laugh were the ones who were readiest to go over the top when the moment came.

Breathing is the most important of our physical functions, in as much as deprivation of air for more than three or four minutes will usually be fatal. We can be without water for four or five days, without food for a month or more. Deep breathing is the most important accessory to vitality on a high plane. If we would have life abundant and flowing over, so that there is reserve for disease conditions and for emergency calls on strength, what we need above all is a copious supply of oxygen, and this can be secured more readily and more easily through laughter than any other way. At the same time the deeper blood oxygenation takes place without anything like the irksomeness of conscious effort that inevitably accompanies definite exercise taken up for its own sake.

When we breathe normally, taking in about five hundred cubic centimetres of air, nearly one-third of that or about 150 c. c. represents what is known as the dead space in the lungs, that is, the air filling the laryngeal cavity, as well as the bronchial tree, for the air filling these parts is not useful in the respiratory process. It is only the air that gets to the alveoli of the lungs, that is, the terminal portions of the bronchi, that actually does respiratory work, bringing about an interchange of oxygen and carbon dioxide between the tissues and the air in the lungs. Of the five hundred cubic centimetres that are breathed in, only about three hundred and fifty are actually made use of in the lungs. Since the vital capacity of the lungs is probably ten times that amount, it is easy to understand that respiratory change may be very slow, and the respiratory process comparatively inactive, unless there is something that sets us breathing deeper. Exercise will do that, and when exercise comes with sport it is very valuable. When it is pursued voluntarily just for the sake of the exercise, it is hard to go on with. But laughter will accomplish the same thoroughgoing stimulation of inspiration as exercise with sport, and it requires no effort of the will at all, but on the contrary, may be accomplished with the greatest pleasure.

How much laughter may mean for deepening breathing is demonstrated very strikingly by what the physiologists say about the ordinary supply of air to the lungs by means of respiration. During a quiet inspiration an adult, as was said, breathes in about five hundred cubic centimetres of air. As a matter of careful observation, however, by very deep inspiration we can breath in some four times that amount. It is very probable that when we laugh even quietly we always breathe in at least twice as much as in ordinary inspiration, and not infrequently in the midst of very hearty laughter, three or four times what is known as the tidal air, that is, the amount breathed in and out in normal, ordinary respiration. The vital capacity of the lungs, that is, the quantity of air that can be breathed out by the deepest possible expiration after making the deepest possible inspiration, is, for the average adult man, over thirty-five hundred cubic centimetres, that is, seven times as much as in quiet breathing. It is very easy to see from this how much laughter may mean in changing the air completely in the lungs, and how much more it accomplishes for complete pulmonary ventilation than ordinary inspiration.

How much the presence of a superabundance of oxygen may mean for making life very different from what it was before was very well illustrated, for fiction purposes at least, by Jules Verne in one of his shorter stories, written some fifty years ago. A distinguished chemist, Dr. Ox, came to the conclusion that if he could only increase the amount of oxygen in the air of a town he could speed up very much the activities of the citizens. He chose a small town in southern Germany where they were noted for the calmness and quietness with which they did things—*Ohne Hast, ohne Rast.* Dinner, for instance, always consumed several hours, and the opera took five or six hours at least, because they were not accustomed to hurrying things. The ingenious doctor had a typically appropriate scene for his experiment. He introduced into the council chamber of the Board of Aldermen so much oxygen, during a session of the Board, that they developed a fad for progress, and decided that the town was too slow and needed "painting up." Dr. Ox secured the contract for the painting, and succeeded in supplying paint continually giving off oxygen. The result was the town began to do things very rapidly. They even revamped a *casus belli* with a neighboring town over a cow that had wandered on to the town common some six hundred years before. They were in the midst of preparations for the war when the amount of oxygen in the air reached a dangerous percentage and there was an explosion, killing only the chief experimenter, and restoring the town to its accustomed peace and quiet and placidity.

Jules Verne's story is, of course, only an impossible romance, exaggerated even beyond his usual custom because it afforded such a good opportunity to the mercurial French for a hearty laugh at their stolid German neighbors. Usually the French romancer studied out very carefully the scientific details of the conditions which he introduced into his stories. It must not be forgotten that as the result of this he anticipated such discoveries as the electric light, the submarine cable, the submarine boat, as well as a number of advances in ballooning and transportation generally. It is not at all unlikely that if it were possible to supply people generally with a greater percentage of oxygen than they secure at the present time, they would have ever so much more incentive and go-aheaditiveness than they have, and they would live their lives on a more active level.

It is clear in a physiological demonstration that laughter brings in this extra supply of oxygen in a perfectly natural way. This surely must have the effect suggested in Jules Verne's story, of stimulating those who indulge in it, and giving them renewed energy and "pep," yet without any deleterious consequences. A great many people who suffer from depression would see that feeling disappear as the result of the more abundant supply of oxygen that would come to them if they made it a point to laugh heartily a number of times every day.

As we shall say a number of times in the course of this book, laughing is largely a habit, and some people actually seem to cultivate the habit of not laughing. There are some families, especially, in which laughs are seldom heard. It is in such families particularly that the psychoneuroses occur by preference. They take themselves too seriously, while those who laugh easily very seldom suffer from the neurotic conditions, which, in our time, seem to be increasing in number, just in proportion as the tendency to laugh quietly, rather than deeply and heartily, is growing. There seems to be a very definite indirect ratio between laughter and the neuroses. The increase of one always means the decrease of the other. If this effect alone can be traced to laughter something of its value as a vital stimulant will be realized.

CHAPTER III

LAUGHTER AND THE HEART

WHILE laughter produces the most direct and immediate effect on the lungs, using them indeed, as the actual medium for the production of most of the phenomena of laughter, it has an almost equally direct and immediate effect on the other important organ of the chest—the heart. The heart is so situated in the thorax that it lies along the diaphragm, its lower part, the right heart, actually resting upon the diaphragm, with only the heart sac, or pericardium, in between the two organs. Almost needless to say, the heart lies much higher in the body than is usually thought. The apex beat, or the point where the apex of the heart impinges on the chest wall, and may be felt, is usually considered to represent the location of the heart. This is, however, the very lowest and outermost part of it. Most actors, when they place their hands on their hearts, especially in connection with exclamations with regard to the heart, set their hands almost exactly over their stomachs.

As the diaphragm is raised and lowered vigorously in hearty laughter, it rubs against the right portion of the heart, and lifts the whole organ up and lets it down more or less rhythmically. This acts as a distinct stimulant to the heart, especially when it is in a healthy condition, and increases both the heart rate, that is, the number of its beats, and also the force of the heartbeat. These effects can be demonstrated any time by counting the pulse just before and after laughter and noting the greater frequency and how much more the pulse wave rises in the arteries against the finger. It is easy to understand under the circumstances that there is a very definite stimulation of the circulation. This is why laughter makes us feel so well and, when heartily indulged in, makes us fairly tingle at the surface of the body.

Such mechanical action upon the heart might possibly be expected to interfere with the heart's activity, or at least to hamper its continuity of action. Experience has shown, however, that it has exactly the opposite effect, and causes the heart to do its work better in every way. Some of the old-fashioned ideas with regard to the heart, and espe-

cially the feeling that the heart represents something else in the body besides the muscle pump that
it really is, persist rather obstinately in a great
many minds.

It is not so long ago in the history of the race
that the heart used to be considered the organ in
which originated love and hate, as well as most of
the other deep and primitive emotions. The heart
was regarded as a very important structure, also, in
the relations it had to thinking. We still continue
to use familiarly, not only in ordinary conversation,
but also in writing, and sometimes even serious
writing, expressions which proclaim these old be-
liefs in the heart as an organ of emotion, if not of
intelligence. We talk, for instance, about a "big-
hearted man," meaning one who takes humanity to
his heart, that is, whose kindly feelings are always
manifest, and who has broad sympathies for all
mankind and their interests. We still talk, also,
about "thinking in the heart" and even about loving
and hating there. Probably no expression from the
Bible is oftener quoted than the well-known sen-
tence, "Only the man who thinketh not in his heart
says there is no God." Archbishop Trench, the
well-known English student of language, spoke of

such modes of expression as fossils in language. Like the fossils that are dug out of the earth, they serve to show what life was in an older time. Our fossil expressions with regard to the heart and its emotional and intellectual activity reveal old-time ideas on the subject, and show very clearly what used to be the prevailing notion as to the significance of the heart in the human body. Almost needless to say, however, we have completely abandoned the notion of the heart as being the origin of anything more than the force which carries on the circulation in the body.

When Steno or Stensen, the distinguished Danish anatomist, after having made the observations which have caused his name to be connected ever since with Steno's duct, the canal that leads the saliva from the parotid glands into the mouth, demonstrated that the heart was only a muscle, his declaration in the matter met with no little opposition from his medical colleagues. Even his previous reputation as a careful original observer did not prove sufficient to obtain a ready hearing for this new and very revolutionary idea. Many people made fun of it, and some of those who did so were educated, and not a few of them were fairly scientific. The notion of the heart as the source of emotions was very deeply entrenched in human thought. As a matter of fact, Steno's work on the subject has not entirely entered into the thought of mankind even yet, and it is the residue of the older ideas as to the heart as the very center of the emotional and intellectual life of man which makes so many people feel that any mechanical irritation of the heart would almost surely do harm rather than good, and might interfere seriously with its activity.

The heart was looked upon as a sort of *noli me tangere*, a touch-me-not, surely not to be interfered with mechanically in any way, or inevitably death would result. We know now, however, that the heart can stand a great deal of physical interference of one kind or another without any serious results following. Stab wounds of the heart have been successfully sewed up, even bullet wounds of it have been recovered from, so that the heart can be depended on to stand severe injury. In a number of cases in animals even perforating bullet wounds of the left heart have not proved fatal. Provided the heart's mechanical activity as a blood pump supplying the rest of the body, and especially the brain, with blood is not interfered with, injuries to the heart may be completely recovered from. It needs no coddling, and irritation, unless carried to an excessive degree, only stimulates it. It is a hardy organ that asks no favors.

The human heart was evidently meant to be stimulated by the various activities of the body. It is a matter of everyday experience that the heart rate increases with muscular exercise. A simple change in posture can affect the heart rate. The rate is higher when standing (80), than when sitting (70), and higher in this latter condition than when lying down (66). Even light muscular work, such as tapping a telegraph key as rapidly as possible, may raise the heart rate from below 70 to over 100 a minute. The effects of moderate or heavy work is correspondingly greater, the pulse rate rising to 150 or even 180 a minute. When the muscular work is continued, the pulse rate rises to a certain maximum which it maintains more or less constantly during the work. Manifestly the heart was meant to be stimulated to higher activity by changes in the body. On the other hand the pulse rate drops very rapidly, reaching the normal in a few seconds on the stoppage of light work, but only

As we work harder the heart must work that much harder.

after a long interval in the case of exhausting muscular work, such as long distance running. There is a most interesting and valuable nervous mechanism, but probably also an essential muscular irritability, which brings about this variation in the heartbeat so as to make it accord with the activities of the body and the needs of the circulation.

Almost needless to say, the heartbeat may vary distinctly with the individual. Some people in perfect health, or at least without having any symptoms over a long life, have very slow hearts, often as low as fifty while sitting down. Napoleon's pulse is said to have been lower even than this, and not to have risen above sixty even in the midst of his battles. On the other hand some persons have a normal pulse beat, even in the reclining position, above eighty, or even ninety, yet remain healthy, and I have myself known one of them live to be nearly seventy-five, and another one well beyond seventy. In both cases death took place not from the heart, but from intercurrent disease. The formula for the heartbeat then is not an absolute one, but depends on a great many circumstances, and it is not surprising to find that there are distinct incidental variations from time to time as well as natural differences.*

In recent years we have learned that in spite of the tradition of supposed supersusceptibility to irritation, so that mechanical disturbance might be fatal, direct heart stimulation encourages that organ to do its work better. Especially is this true when, because of lack of exercise, the heart has become lazy as it were, or is doing its work inadequately. When people feel faint, or feel as if they were going to, it is now well-known that having them swallow a series of small sips of water, or, for that matter, any other fluid, is rather an effective way of reviving them. The actual swallowing movement has a direct mechanical effect on the heart for the esophagus, or swallowing tube, passes close to that organ, and the process of swal-

---

* It seems to be determined that the taller the individual, the slower his pulse. There is said to be a constant relationship in this matter, and a definite mathematical formula has been worked out. It might possibly be expected that the larger man, on account of the extent of his circulation, would require a higher pulse beat, but the opposite is true. The same rule holds among the animals of different species. Small animals, as a rule, have a higher pulse rate than larger ones. Thus, elephants have a pulse rate of 25 to 28 a minute, the horse and ox, 35 to 50, the sheep, 60 to 80, the dog, 100 to 120, the rabbit, 150, and mice 700. Buchanan says the canary heart beats at the rate of 1,000 per minute.

lowing probably acts directly on the heart structure. This stimulates the heart's vitality and sets
it going more actively again, when for any reason
it has become sluggish. It is not the fluid itself,
but it is the act of swallowing and its repetition
a number of times which, by the massage exerted
by the swallowing movement on the heart muscle,
wakes the heart up to renewed activity. Nature
has a series of such tricks up her sleeve.

It is a common experience with animals in the
physiological laboratory that when for some reason
the heart stops beating, it can usually be restored
to renewed activity by direct massage of the heart
muscle. In this way an animal whose heart would
not again have taken up beating if left to itself—
and failure to beat would mean death—may be
raised to life again, as it were, and completely recover. It has even been suggested that in abdominal operations when, as the result of the anæsthetic,
or of shock, the heart stops beating, which happens
very rarely, though it is occasionally seen, the
surgeon should put his hand directly under the
heart beneath the diaphragm and push upward in
such a way as to produce direct mechanical irritation of the heart in order to set it going once

more. I believe that in some cases this maneuver has been found very valuable, and even successful in restoring to life patients whose hearts had stopped, and who might, as a consequence of this, have failed to come to. Direct heart stimulation has proved life saving.

Mechanical action upon the heart, then, has come to be looked upon as a valuable agent in the stimulation of its activity and the restoration of function. While people with neurotic heart conditions may feel a little anxious about the possible deleterious effect of laughter on their hearts, complete reassurance has come in that matter, and in addition, the feeling that undoubtedly laughter represents an excellent heart stimulant for this class of hearts. People who suffer from missed pulse beat, extra systole as it is called, probably get more relief for their uncomfortable consciousness of their heart action through laughter than in any other way. I have known them, after they had been worrying for days lest their heart should stop for good, to go to a good lively farce comedy and laugh themselves into a state of absolute good feeling that would last for some days. Indeed, I know nothing that has such favorable action on this form of heart trouble as the cultivation of the habit of hearty laughing. The movement of the diaphragm acts above all upon the right heart, and as this is thin walled, and particularly the auricle on the right side is quite thin, the action of the diaphragm on the heart must be quite definite and positive. It is in this right side of the heart, as recent investigations of cardiac activity have shown, that the cycle of the heartbeat begins, so that stimulation of the auricular area might very well prove excellent for the renewal of heart activity, and especially for its regularization when there is a functional irregularity.

It might be thought that such stimulation would mean very little, since the heart is presumably dependent on the central nervous system, and acts as a result of impulses that are conveyed to it without any question of the heart muscle itself influencing its own movement primarily. This idea, though rather commonly entertained, is distinctly in opposition to the known physiology of the heart's action. The heartbeat is one of our unconscious activities, which goes on as well when we are asleep as during our waking hours. There are other unconscious activities, as respiration and peristalsis, that is, the regular, wavelike motion in the intestines, and certain other functions that are performed under like conditions of absence of attention, so far as the nervous system associated with consciousness is concerned. These are controlled by the lower central and sympathetic nervous systems. The heart might easily be expected to operate the same way in rather thoroughgoing dependence on the nervous system, and in that case mechanical irritation could not be expected to influence it to any extent.

While the heart is dependent on the nervous system for its regulation, there being inhibitory fibers which keep it from going too fast, and accelerator fibers which keep it from going too slowly, very much as the governor of a steam engine acts, its essential muscular activity is primary and not secondary. As a matter of fact the heart is the *primum movens* in the body, that is to say, it is the first structure in the organism which demonstrates by its activity that life is present and producing motion. In the chick, as studied in the embryo, that is, the white spot in the egg when germination has begun, it is noted that very early in the development of the animal, long before the nervous system has begun to develop, the material out of which the heart is to take form a little later, begins to pulsate at regular intervals. Once this starts its motion, it continues until the end of life, and any cessation means death. Life and death here come closest.

This is the demonstration that the heart has within itself its own central activity. It is possessed of spontaneous motility, that is, its motion comes from something intrinsic and not something extrinsic. It is only a muscle pump, but it runs of itself. Irritation of it causes such reaction as leads to higher vital activity, and this is very well effected by means of laughter. The jerky movements of the diaphragm serve to irritate it physiologically and not pathologically and the result is stimulation.*

When one is feeling "downhearted" as the expression is or when the trials of life have "taken the heart out of us" or "discouraged" us, which, etymo-

---

* Dr. Carrel's experiment, at the Rockefeller Institute, with the portion of excised chicken heart which has been beating for some ten years after the death of the organism to which it originally belonged, is only another demonstration of the essential quality of the heart's action and of the fact that there is something in the heart itself that causes it.

logically, is only another way of saying the same thing, laughter will do more to set the heart going regularly and properly again than anything else. It may not always be easy to secure this action, because, unfortunately, the desire for laughter may be absent, but it must not be forgotten that laughter is largely a habit, like a great many other things, and that it may be cultivated to good advantage. Some people seem to make it a rule of life not to laugh any more than they absolutely have to, while others laugh on every possible occasion. These latter people not only enjoy life more, but they actually have more physical energy to dispose of, and their organs accomplish their functions better.

All of our deepest feelings have a special action on the heart. As a result we have been accustomed to talk about various dislocations of that organ, and we have the expression that "the heart was in the mouth," or felt to be "way down in our boots," and these are picturesque descriptions of the feelings that we experience. They represent functional affections of the heart that can, as a rule, be influenced favorably by laughter. They represent the feeling that the heart is not in its place, but is somewhere else. Laughter gives one the feeling of bringing the heart back to its place.*

It must not be forgotten that even where there is serious degeneration of the heart affecting also the muscle, the entrance of a physician into

---

* A good story comes from the Civil War which illustrates this very well. It may be a fable *se non é vero é ben trovato:* Two soldiers in the Union Army, one of them an Irishman and the other a colored man, were, by the curious coincidence that sometimes occurs, wounded exactly in the same way. The bullet hit them just over the heart, but by a very fortunate chance glanced on the rib and ricocheted, that is, skipped somewhat as a flat stone will on the surface of water, around the chest, along the rib to the back and there made its exit. The wound of entrance and exit of the bullet were almost exactly opposite each other, and the only thing that a casual observer could think was that here was a bullet wound directly through the heart. There were a great many wounded, and the facilities for caring for them were overtaxed, so when the stretcher bearers got to the Irishman they were about to leave him for dead, or hopelessly wounded, thinking it was not worth while trying to do anything for him, but he came to as they talked over him and insisted that he was at least as good as three dead men yet. When next day he proved to be in such good condition that he was evidently on the high road to get better, the surgeon asked him how it was that he was not dead since the bullet seemed almost inevitably to have gone right through his heart. His reply was, "Sure when I was struck we were just beginning the attack and my heart was in my mouth." The colored soldier had exactly the same sort of wound, and he too began to recover as soon as he reached the hospital. When the surgeon asked him how it was that he was not killed he replied, "Oh, Doctor, they were just attacking us when I was hit, and my heart was in my boots." Perhaps these may be the racial peculiarities as to dislocation of the heart under these circumstances, even though the organ may not go to the extent represented by the expressions.

the sick room with a placid smile which puts confidence into the patient, will make his heart activity much better. Even under these circumstances a smile is contagious, and while it may not be accompanied by any special movement of the diaphragm, the effect upon the mind is reflected in the heart to the patient's benefit. Many a heart specialist has owed his reputation for always doing his heart patients good to the fact that he had a contagious smile that lifted them out of the sense of depression that was coming over them. No organ of the body is so likely to produce depression of spirits so readily as a heart that is affected in any way. The English rule with regard to angina is that the more fuss that is made about it, the less serious is the actual pathological condition. When there is a great deal of complaint, it is not true angina. Something of the same thing is true with regard to depression consequent upon heart trouble. The depression that is deepest is very often the result of some functional heart trouble, or perhaps, functional heart trouble grafted on a definite pathological condition that is not in itself very serious. It is under these circumstances that anything that will bring good cheer to the patient will almost surely make a very great difference in his condition.

Joyous feelings are, as a rule, even more influential in their action upon the heart than the depressive feelings or the panicky dreads. Physicians know only too well that a great feeling of joy may be as serious for a weak-hearted patient as a scare or a shock. We have to be careful when near relatives, who have not been seen for many years, are to be introduced into the sick room of delicate patients, because we must break the joyful news to them gently, as well as the sorrowful.

In a word, the heart is deeply under the influence of the emotions, and the emotional quality of laughter, combined with its mechanical effect upon the heart, does a great deal to stimulate that organ to accomplish its purposes to the very best degree. The great majority of people, especially after middle life, do not laugh nearly enough for the good of their hearts. Many of them would feel ever so much better if they indulged freely in laughter, and thus aroused the heart into a renewal of its activities on the highest plane. The prescription seems too easy to be of any very great value, but it is the little things in human nature that count. There are secretions of glands so minute that the amount which the body receives in a day is so small as to be scarcely measurable by the most careful chemical research, and yet without it life is either impossible or very much disturbed.

CHAPTER IV

LAUGHTER AND THE LIVER

THE liver is by far the largest and the heaviest organ in the body, weighing nearly one-thirtieth of the body weight. It is not surprising then to find that it is an extremely important organ for health, and that any disturbance of it is likely to produce rather serious results, though they may be only passing, and that on the other hand, anything that stimulates it to perform its functions better may mean a great deal for the relief of disturbing symptoms of various kinds. It probably must be considered the most essential organ in the abdominal region, far more significant than other organs of which we hear more. We used to think of it as being, in a certain sense, an excretory organ, that it is to say, as the portal system of circulation carries the blood from the intestines directly into the liver, and bile is manufactured there, it was concluded that this substance was something that had been removed from the blood because it was not wholesome for the rest of the body. Whenever this material was reabsorbed into the system, people became bilious, and suffered from a number of very disturbing symptoms, while melancholia, as the etymology of the word indicates, is the demonstration that the ancients thought that extreme depression of mind was due to the presence of "black bile" absorbed into the system.

We know now, however, that the bile is an extremely valuable secretion manufactured by the liver to aid in the digestion of food. We used to think that most of the digestion was done in the stomach, and now we know that the stomach is scarcely more than the enlarged end of the swallowing tube, meant to retain food for a time, in order that the intestines may not be overloaded, and then pass it on at regular intervals for ultimate effective digestion in the intestines. The stomach, as we shall see, saves us from having to spend the better part of our time eating, as so many of the animals do. The most important digestive organ of the body is the liver, which pours its secretion into the portion of the intestines known as the duodenum, very slightly below the pylorus, or gateway from the stomach to the intestines. Just as soon as food finds its way into the intestine, nervous reflexes cause a flow of bile, and the process of digestion is seriously taken up. The bile contains a series of ferments, especially an important fat-splitting ferment, probably a protein-dissolving ferment, and it also contains some very interesting antiseptic substances which prevent the growth of deleterious microörganisms in the intestinal tract. No wonder that any disturbance of the flow of bile, or especially any back flow of it into the stomach, will produce quite seriously disturbing symptoms.

Nature in her economy always provides for more than one function in an organ, and very often combines, in the same organic structure, a series of functions. The liver, besides being an extremely important digestive organ because of the secretion it pours into the intestines, is also a ductless gland, or at least of an analagous nature to a ductless gland, and has a good deal to do with the manufacture of glycogen, or muscle sugar, out of starchy material. The liver has been demonstrated to be a storehouse of this material, and from here it is poured into the circulation and deposited in the muscles, or burned up in them to provide muscle energy as it is needed. When soldiers are to travel light, and yet go long distances and retain their energy, the best concentrated food for them is candy or sugar. In recent wars, just as far as possible, sugar and candy have been served to the troops, especially in times of critical emergencies when much is expected of them, and regular meals might be delayed. Athletic coaches have come to recognize the value of sugar for intense muscle effort. It is said that one of the recent English university boat races proved such a reversal of form because shortly before the race one of the crews was given a very liberal allowance of sugar to eat. This was a sort of experiment, but it worked wonders, and the crew proved fresh, as winners four lengths ahead, though their opponents were fainting in their boats.

It is not surprising then that interference with liver functions very soon brings with it serious disturbance of health. The old-fashioned, popular idea of a sluggish liver probably has a definite scientific significance even at the present time, after the accumulation of an immense amount of information with regard to the liver in recent years. The presence of biliary materials and especially the bile salts in the intestines is important for the encouragement of peristalsis and therefore for the proper evacuation of waste material. Constipation used to be said to be due largely to a sluggish liver, and the use of bile salts certainly relieves it promptly. Sluggish livers are often said to occur particularly in those who do not get out in the air much, and who do not take much exercise. There seems no doubt that exercise has a good deal to do with stimulating the function of the liver. This is accomplished partly by the call made on the liver for further supplies of glycogen whenever the muscles are actively used, but mainly because of the direct mechanical stimulation of the liver which occurs in connection with the taking of exercise. This is rather easy to understand, though its significance has apparently been missed to a very great extent. The liver's position in the body, and its inevitable tendency to be affected by movements of the diaphragm and of the abdominal muscles make it very clear how much exercise must affect it.

The four to six pounds of rather solid material which constitutes the liver hang somewhat free in the abdominal cavity, supported by ligaments, some of which have an anchorage on the abdominal wall, and some of them on the diaphragm. It is easy to understand that whenever we run or move rapidly, or whenever we jump, or go up and down stairs, the liver is moved rather freely, and there must be a good deal of stimulation of its circulation. Jumping particularly stirs up the liver rather roughly, but manifestly that fits in with the purposes of nature, and the irritation is a stimulant to function rather than a disturbance.

As people grow older, however, they very seldom run and they jump almost never, so that the principal exercise for the liver is the rather mild shaking up that comes in connection with walking. Of course, if a man is engaged in an occupation that requires a good deal of stooping and bending, his liver comes to be massaged a good deal between the thoracic and abdominal contents, and their muscle walls, so that the circulation in it is well stimulated. As a rule, however, men do not indulge in this sort of activity to any extent as the years advance. No wonder there is the complaint of sluggish liver in the older folk. The liver evidently does its work better under conditions in which it receives considerable shaking about.

Laughing, however, produces a very definite ef-

fect on the liver. Its influence is very easy to
understand if the anatomical relations of the liver
are recalled. The liver is situated in the right
upper quadrant of the abdomen, immediately
underneath the diaphragm, the upper curvature of
the liver causing the diaphragm to arch upward
more on the right side than it does on the left.
As the diaphragm goes down, and it often descends
three or four or more inches, at the margins, and
probably six to seven inches at the dome of the
midriff, the liver is carried down by it and then
up again with the upward excursion of the diaphragm. This gives rise to a distinct massage of
the liver which is excellent for the stimulation of
its circulation and of its functions.

Altogether we manufacture twenty or more
ounces of bile in the day, which performs an important function in the digestion of food. It is
said that some people whose liver functions are not
very active, somehow manage to get along with
about one-half of this, but of course their digestion
is not accomplished so thoroughly or so satisfactorily. Hence the number of liver stimulants of
one kind or another that are sold. The extensive
advertisement of them would seem to indicate that

a large percentage of our people need help for the proper performance of liver function. The bile will be produced without any artificial stimulation if the liver is properly stimulated, but it will not if there is no massage or rubbing of it to encourage circulation through it, and keep functions active. Exercise in the young, laughter in those who are older and whose dignity will not permit them to make hurried movements, are necessary for proper liver functioning.

Liver secretion is very like salivary secretion. We manufacture, if there is call for it in the mouth, some twenty ounces of saliva in the twenty-four hours. The presence of food in the mouth, or even on the plate before us, if it is appetizing, will cause saliva to flow, hence our expression that something we like to eat "makes the mouth water." The amount of saliva which will be secreted depends very largely after this preliminary excitation not on the amount of food we take, but on the amount of chewing that we do. If our food is prepared for us, as it is unfortunately in the modern time, in such a way that we have to do very little chewing, then mastication will be limited—for we never do anything unless we have to—and we shall have a correspondingly small amount of saliva. Some people are said not to use much more than one-half the normal amount of saliva in the day. This is the reason why the teeth of mankind are so bad in our time, for we have the cook do all the chewing for us, and nearly everything is served so soft that a minimum amount of mastication is needed. The lack of saliva is a serious thing for mouth conditions. All the highly advertised tooth pastes and tooth washes announce that they correct the acidity of the mouth which causes caries of the teeth, and predisposes to pyorrhea, but the salivary secretion is, under normal conditions, strongly alkaline, and is the best possible corrective of that unfortunate acidity of the mouth which is causing so much damage to the teeth in our time.

Unfortunately our salivary glands are not called upon to manufacture enough saliva. Much more of it would be secreted into the mouth if food materials were more vigorously chewed. Mankind will not chew much unless it has to. There is no use preaching mastication unless the food is tougher and requires it. An older generation used harder materials, that is, tougher foods that demanded more chewing, and thus they protected their teeth much better than we do at the present time, in spite of all our dentists and our dentifrices and the rest. At the same time they secreted more of the valuable digestive juice.

Something very like this is happening with regard to the bile. We need exercise and massage of the liver so as to have a more abundant flow of bile. That is why mankind has always made mealtime, as a rule, a period of jollity, and why, if men and women sit around after a meal, they are prone to laugh a good deal. A sense of stomach repletion tempts to laughter, as we have said. Laughter, by its up and down movements of the diaphragm, causes a good deal of massage of the liver, stimulates its activity and undoubtedly brings about a greater flow of bile. This favors more complete digestion of food, better absorption and metabolism of food materials, and its presence in notable quantities stimulates peristalsis, and therefore brings about regular evacuation of the bowels, which is extremely important for health.

Laughing becomes a very important adjunct of digestion under these circumstances. Men have always known that fun and jollity after meals were good for digestion and health in general, but they have not realized the exact physiological conditions which brought about the improvement in digestion.

This has come to us with the recognition of the rôle of laughter in stimulating the liver and other digestive organic functions. As we shall see, there is stimulation of the stomach and pancreas, as well as of the liver, and this also undoubtedly aids digestion. The liver, however, being a very large and heavy organ that is carried up and down with the excursions of the diaphragm, its massage secures more and more of the beneficial effect of laughter on digestion. This comes through liver agitation better than in any other way.

The gall bladder, which is an important adjunct to the liver, used to be thought a reservoir for the storage of bile until it should be needed. The old idea of its function was that, in the intervals between digestion, bile gradually accumulated in the gall bladder in order to be ready for the next meal. As a normal gall bladder holds only six to eight drams, that is something less than an ounce, and as eight ounces or more of bile may be secreted in the course of an hour or so during the height of digestion, it would not seem that this amount of storage capacity would be very valuable in facilitating biliary function. In recent years it has come to be felt that very probably the gall bladder serves to maintain a certain pressure on the liver cells, and that this is the real purpose of it. In that case it becomes easy to understand how laughter, by jolting the liver, and so stimulating it, may prove to be very valuable, especially after meals, when bile is needed in quantities for digestion. For these movements act upon the gall bladder and stimulate its pressure function.

One thing is perfectly sure, that those who laugh with and after their meals are much more likely to have good digestion, and to be free from various inconveniences that are associated with indigestion, than those who do not practice the same salutary habit. The old health maxim, "Laugh and grow fat," probably has more meaning in connection with the liver than any other organ, for it is the liver which secretes the principal fat-splitting ferment by which the fat is prepared in such a way in the intestines that it may be absorbed and assimilated into the human system. Fat is not directly absorbed, but is changed from the particular animal fat or plant fat that it consists of into that special fatty material which characterizes the human being. In a word, a whole series of the most important functions of digestion connected with the liver and its secretion are surely stimulated to higher activity by the liver massage which inevitably occurs in association with hearty laughter.

During these past few years an extremely important discovery has been made in medicine, greatly increasing the significance of the liver and emphasizing all that has been said here as to the value of massage of it. It has been found that patients suffering from the severe forms of anemia, even those extreme anemic conditions which, when fatal, have been called pernicious anemia, are often greatly relieved, and sometimes completely cured, by the administration of liver extract, or even by the taking of ordinary liver substance in the diet. These affections were so serious and usually, indeed, so fatal, that it is easy to understand how important this discovery has proved, for the severe anemias were constantly increasing in number, and the cause of them was absolutely unknown. It seems very probable that this indicates that there is an internal secretion of the liver, or some ingredient ordinarily manufactured by the liver, which is important for the healthy constitution of the blood. Whether this ingredient might not be made to flow more freely into the blood stream as the result of the rather vigorous massage of the liver which comes in connection with hearty laughter remains to be demonstrated, but certainly it would seem as though the stimulation of the circulation, which is thus brought about, would surely be helpful for patients of this kind, and also for all anemic patients where there is any possibility of the liver factor being important in them.

CHAPTER V

LAUGHTER AND THE PANCREAS

AFTER the liver, in close anatomical relation with it, there is a second organ which is situated just below the diaphragm, which is undoubtedly affected to a noteworthy extent by the up and down excursions of the diaphragm during laughter. This is the pancreas, an organ that up to this time has not been at all well known by the generality of people, though physicians in recent years have come to realize that it is an extremely important part of the human anatomy. It forms a long narrow gland reaching from the spleen to the curvature of the duodenum, which lies in intimate anatomical relations with the liver. Its main duct opens into the duodenum, that is, the portion of the small intestine reaching for twelve fingers in breadth—hence the name—from the opening out of the stomach into the intestines. The main bile duct and that of the pancreas often terminate by a common opening some two inches beyond the pylorus, or gateway of the stomach.

After the liver, this is by far the most important digestive organ that we have, for the pancreas has three very important digestive operations to perform. It secretes *trypsin* which digests protein material, that is, lean meat and the body-building materials generally, besides a diastasic enzyme, *amylase*, which digests and prepares starchy food for absorption, and finally it has a fat-digesting ferment *lipase* or *steapsin*, which enables us to digest and absorb fat, for fat is not merely absorbed, but a definite change is produced in it by the digestive organs of different animals that enables them to deposit the particular kind of fat to be found in their tissues no matter what the form of fat may be that they have eaten. The pancreas therefore has much to do with the digestion of all the most valuable classes of food materials.

The importance of the secretion of the pancreas will be best appreciated from the fact that the average amount of pancreatic fluid in the day is about the same as that of the bile from the liver, though the liver would seem to be, because of its size and weight, a much more significant organ. Any serious injury or disease of the pancreas is almost inevitably followed by death. Tumors of the pancreas are almost surely fatal, and cancer of it is always fatal. It is an organ of no great consistency, one of those that, in animals, are called by the butchers the sweetbreads. It is easy to understand, then, that laughter would have very definite direct effect on it, because movements of the diaphragm must be felt all through these rather loosely connected bundles of cells, which are situated where the diaphragmatic movements are greatest, in the immediate neighborhood of the stomach.

Besides its external secretion, however, the pancreas has an internal secretion, that is to say, certain glandular cells in it manufacture a substance which is poured directly into the blood, and does not find its way into the pancreatic ducts, and thence to the intestines. This substance is secreted in extremely minute quantities, but it is intensely active and is very valuable for health, and above all for the maintenance of muscular strength. Its active principle is represented by insulin which was first isolated a few years ago at the University of Toronto by Drs. Banting and Ross. A generation before their discovery, it had been realized that any pathological disturbance of the pancreas which affected the interior of the gland, that is the portions of it known, because of their discoverer, as the islands of Langerhans, brought about diabetes. Insulin is so called after the Latin word *insula*, which means an island, because of the connection between the secretion and these pancreatic islands. Diabetes used to be attributed to various other organs, notably the kidneys and the liver, but the pancreatic element in its causation is now very well determined. There is a substance manufactured by the pancreas, and which gets into the blood stream, that is indispensable for enabling the human body to use up sugar in various metabolic processes. The sugar in the form of glycogen is burned in the muscles in the production of the heat and energy which must develop in connection with muscular movements.

If there is no pancreatic internal secretion for this purpose of making blood sugar properly available in the muscles, the sugar which finds its way from the blood into the liver, but is not in a form in which it can be used up readily, is eliminated by the kidneys as a useless substance, as, under the circumstances, a waste material. This is what constitutes diabetes, or at least glycosuria.

This disease has been increasing very much in recent years in about a direct ratio with the decrease of exercise and the increased consumption of sugary materials. Diabetes is nearly ten times as common now as it used to be a generation ago, and even at the present time, in spite of the discovery of insulin, it still causes a large number of deaths, and is a distinct factor in the mortality lists. Above all its presence often proves very depressing, and not a few of the suicides of people in middle life are due to the disease. It produces great weakness at first, and makes the sufferer from it liable to infections of various kinds, so that he develops boils or carbuncles rather easily, and is particularly prone to suffer from tuberculosis if he is exposed to the contagion of the disease. After a time moreover, gangrene may occur or coma may develop, and the eyesight may be lost by cataract and other serious symptoms may be noted.

It is extremely important therefore to have the pancreas do its work well. It is a rather soft organ lying just below the diaphragm, and it is very clear that as the diaphragm goes up and down in laughter it must be rather vigorously massaged. All the organs in the abdomen have certain contacts with each other, or with cushions of fat that surround them, so that any movement that occurs sets all the organs going to some extent, and hearty laughter must produce a good many movements. This massaging of the pancreas, especially after meals, undoubtedly leads to the manufacture of more of its external secretion, and this makes digestion in the small intestine proceed more vigorously.

The massage of the pancreas, however, probably increases the circulation in the organ, and this stimulates the vital activity of the cells of the pancreas and leads to the production of more of the internal secretion. Diabetes occurs particularly in connection with obesity, and while fat people, that is, those somewhat above weight, are good laughers, the obese often take themselves very seriously and seem to find it too much of an effort to laugh heartily. Some of them actually would be able to laugh their "corporation" away if they could be made to laugh enough. The stout people who are good hearty laughers suffer from diabetes ever so much more rarely than the glum and serious people. This fact has only been noted in recent years in connection with the increase of diabetes in both seriousness and frequency. It has been noted also that worry is a great preliminary condition for diabetes. After a man has gone through a serious business crisis, or a high-pitched political campaign, his diabetes is likely to be ever so much worse. It has even been noted that there is a definite tendency to much less laughter than before in these men, and it is probable that this has much to do with the deterioration of their condition. The diabetes itself has a true pathological etiology, that is, a real disease condition as its basis, but the functional symptoms are rendered much worse because of the lack of the stimulation of the pancreas by the decrease in the amount of laughter.

Little things of this kind mean a very great deal for health, and it has often been very hard to trace the connection of cause and effect in these cases, but with a study of the diaphragm, and its anatomical relations, and its activity in laughter, it becomes very much easier to understand how functional disturbances of digestion and absorption of food materials are connected directly with the decrease in laughter that is so often noted in these patients.

CHAPTER VI

LAUGHTER AND THE SPLEEN AND
DUCTLESS GLANDS

THERE are a series of organs, some of them in intimate relations with the diaphragm, and others situated at various parts of the organism, that may be affected directly by laughter, or indirectly through the increased blood supply to them. The most interesting feature of a number of these organs is that for a while they were considered by the physiologists and actually called by the anatomists "useless" organs. Medical scientists did not know their functions, and because they did not know them, being quite sure that if there had been any use for them they would know it, they called them useless organs. Among them are such important organs as the spleen, and the thyroid, and the suprarenal bodies or glands, not to mention a number of smaller structures situated at various parts of the system. The spleen can be removed without causing the death of the individual, and therefore it was considered to be useless, but the fact that the bone marrow from being yellow turns to red and becomes "splenified" as a compensatory reaction when the spleen is removed, shows how nature can make up for the loss of even an important organ.

Because of the lack of knowledge of the purpose of these organs, and their denomination "useless," it was said that they represented vestiges from preceding stages of evolution, which were no longer of service to the system and were in process of disappearing. Dozens of these organs were described, and they were proclaimed to represent almost unanswerable arguments in support of the theory of evolution. It is something of a joke on the overanxious biologists that subsequent study has made it very clear that many of these organs supposed to be useless are now counted among the most important in the body. Some of them are absolutely essential to life. A few of them at least furnish secretions, which, though in but minimum quantities, affect deeply the mental as well as the physical life. They are now the most interesting organs in the body, and more theories of disease causation and of the cure of various affections are founded on them than on any other organs of the body. Anything that affects them even slightly is sure to produce rather definite alterations in body function and to affect health rather deeply.

The function of the spleen is not well understood, but the most definite facts learned about the organ in recent years are in connection with its movements. It has been shown that there is a marked expansion and contraction of that organ which takes place synchronously with the digestion period. After a meal the spleen begins to increase in size, reaching a maximum at about the fifth hour, and then slowly returns to its previous size. In addition to this slow movement, of expansion and contraction, there is a rhythmical contraction and relaxation of the organ occurring at short intervals, but quite regularly. These frequent movements are supposed to be intended to maintain the circulation through the spleen, and that makes this organ unique among the organs of the body, for none of the others has such a local arrangement for maintaining its circulation. It is easy to understand that these movements of the spleen are stimulated by the up and down movements of the diaphragm, for the spleen is situated immediately beneath the diaphragm, occupying a corresponding position on the left side to that of the liver on the right side. The splenic circulation has much to do with the distribution of iron through the body, and while we have only a very small amount of iron, that is extremely important, for the oxygen carrier in the red blood corpuscles is an iron salt, which oxidizes and deoxidizes very readily.

The spleen has much to do with blood making, and the blood has been coming more and more into prominence as an adjuvant for health and for recovery from disease in recent years. Blood transfusion has become ever so much commoner than it used to be, and undoubtedly gives renewed life to the patient. Massage of the spleen, then, because of its blood-making function, represents an extremely important factor for the health of the body. The spleen is of rather soft consistency so that movements of the diaphragm in its neighborhood must influence the circulation in the organ rather notably. It has been suggested that in tropical countries it is too warm during most of the year to indulge either in exercise or in very hearty laughter, so that perhaps this is one of the reasons why splenic enlargement occurs so much more frequently in the tropics, though undoubtedly in many of these cases some infectious element is present. The spleen's relation to digestion, that is, stomach digestion, and its rhythmic contractions in close relationship with those of the stomach, make the rôle of laughter in relation to the spleen even more significant than would otherwise be the case. We shall discuss in the following chapter the effect of laughter on the stomach, and its correspondence with the spleen should be noted.

There are other ductless glands, however, that are brought into rather intimate touch with the diaphragm in its excursions in laughter. These are the suprarenal glands, about the size and shape of the little finger crooked in its last two joints. These organs lie just above the kidneys on each side, hence their name. The upper pole of the right kidney is pressed upon by the liver, fitting into a depression in that organ as we have said. It is easy to understand how between these two organs the suprarenal on this side is massaged to no slight degree during movements of the diaphragm that carry the liver up and down. The suprarenal on the left side is caught between the kidney and the diaphragm, slightly at least, and so it is rubbed, if not massaged, when the deeper movements of the diaphragm take place.

These movements undoubtedly arouse the suprarenals into higher functional activity, bring more blood to them, and therefore cause more of their secretion to find its way into the circulation. The secretion of the suprarenals is extremely important for health. It tones the muscular coat of the blood vessels and also the heart muscles, raises blood pressure, and as a consequence makes the man who feels "down in the dumps" pick himself up and feel, as one man said, "like a million dollars." Indeed, very probably a good deal of the effect of laughter on the disposition, lifting it up from grave to gay, is due to the influence of the excursions of the diaphragm upon the suprarenals during the process.

How important the secretion of the suprarenals is will be best understood from the fact that disease of the suprarenals, Addison's disease as it is called, from the distinguished English physician who was the first to describe it, is invariably fatal. It is accompanied by great reduction in blood pressure, and deposit of pigment at various irritated parts of the body, as the tongue, the waistline, and the wrists, apparently as the result of the lowered blood pressure. Great weakness results also from the lowered pressure, so that the patient is scarcely able to drag himself about, and to the intensification of this weakness the patient eventually succumbs. The amount of suprarenal substance that is needed to maintain the tone of the arteries and, through that, normal blood pressure, is almost infinitesimal. It is represented by a very high decimal fraction of the body weight, but trifling as it would seem to be, it is absolutely essential for health and strength and the continuance of life.

Addison's disease is usually due to tuberculosis of the suprarenals and the tubercle bacillus has a definite tendency to implantation in tissues that are inactive, or in which the circulation is somewhat defective. It is easy to understand how the up and down movements of the diaphragm rubbing upon the suprarenals might very well prevent that slowing up of the circulation which favors the implantation of the tubercle bacilli. These mechanical factors in the conservation of health and the prevention of disease have not been given as much weight as they deserve because physicians have been inclined to be more occupied with the chemical treatment of them. Laughter is, however, one of the most important of them, and undoubtedly produces good effect.

It would take but very little stimulation of the suprarenal glands to produce very important effects in various bodily functions. If laughter had but minimal efficacy in the increase of blood supply to these organs, the systemic result would be very striking. Certainly the diaphragm cannot make the large excursions and the jerky movements connected with laughter without having some effect, and even the slightest would be far-reaching in its modification of a number of important bodily functions.

There is another important portion of the body in which laughter produces very definite effects upon the ductless glands. This is the cervical region, that is, the neck. Any one who will hold his hand over his neck while he laughs heartily will note at once what rather large vibrations are set up in all the neck structures. The thrill of them is felt in the hand and it is easy to understand that there is a good deal of massage-like effect produced by this vibration, which is due to the outrush of air through the trachea, and the deep respirations to replace it, but above all, the sounds made in the larynx and vocal cords as the laughter continues.

These cervical vibrations undoubtedly influence the circulation to all the structures in the neck. In recent years a number of different kinds of vibratory instruments have been designed for massage purposes, especially for the face and neck, but none of them is equal to laughter in the effect that is produced, not merely on the skin, but on the deeper structures. Here in the neck region there is a series of ductless glands that are of very great significance for health and some of which are essential to life. Here we have the thyroid gland, and the thymus in early life, as well as its remains later, and we have never been quite able to assure ourselves that even the atrophied remnant of the thymus that is left is not of definite importance for some physiological purpose in the system. In addition there are the parathyroid glands, small bodies situated at the sides of the neck and bearing certain relations to the thyroid, but evidently quite independent of it. Besides there are certain small glandular bodies in connection with the blood vessels of the neck, the so-called carotid glands or bodies, the real meaning of which is not very clear as yet, though we are inclined to think of them as representing important endocrine tissues since so many of the other mysterious organs of unknown function have proved to be ever so much more important than we dreamed a few years ago.

The thyroid is so important that the absence of its secretion means almost inevitable death. The removal of the whole thyroid is sure to be fatal. It supplies iodine for the system, and iodine is absolutely essential to life, but it seems also to be essential for intelligence. It is said that only about four hundred-thousandths of a grain of iodine a day is needed for the metabolism, but without that much man becomes a blithering idiot and if he is entirely deprived of it, death ensues.

Removal of all the parathyroid bodies invariably brings about certain deep-seated nervous symptoms and a fatal termination. We have not been able to find just what their physiological significance is, except that their removal is followed by tetany and death. They regulate nervous control in some very important way so that stimulation of them must produce very definite effects.

The carotid glands, lying along the carotid

arteries, are others of this group of glandular structures which exist in the neck and which are subjected to vibratory massage during laughter. No very vehement effect is produced on them, but just enough to encourage circulation through them and therefore stimulate their secretion.

We have come to realize that these ductless glands mean ever so much for health and strength, and for euphoria, or good feeling. Weight for weight, they are by far the most important structures in the body. They represent the most important factors in the chemistry of the body. As time goes on these organs, which for a time were considered to be more or less useless, and indeed, most of them were counted among the vestigial structures in the body—the purpose of which had been outlived, though the organs remained to do harm rather than good—are actually the most useful that we have.

A great many physicians in our time are very much inclined to think that the most important scientific development in modern medicine has come with regard to our increase of knowledge of the significance to the body of the ductless glands or endocrines, as they have come to be called. Not a few physicians are inclined to attribute a number of the functional disturbances of health to deficiency of endocrine secretion or the occurrence of endocrine imbalance. As a result a very definite effort has been made to employ for such deficiencies the extracts or active principles, or sometimes even the crude substance of the ductless glands of animals. We are flooded with preparations to compensate for this endocrine disturbance in the human body, but I need scarcely say that their efficacy is considered very dubious. We need only extremely minute quantities of the secretions of the ductless glands to regulate our economy. Any excess of these is sure to produce quite serious effects. The glandular products have been used so unwittingly that probably it is very fortunate that nature knows how to prevent anything like an excess of endocrine material in the system. If many of the animal products in this line were actually active they would represent massive doses where only the minutest quantities are needed.

Laughter by its action through the circulation, and because of the gentle massage of ductless glands that is associated with it, promises to use nature's own methods of stimulating the ductless glands, and thus increasing their natural secretion. Careful observations have shown that states of mind influence the ductless glands profoundly. Especially is this true as regards the suprarenals and the thyroid, and such mental conditions as worry or anger or fear or terror may greatly affect the amount of secretion given off by them. More cheerful moods have an opposite effect, and relieve the body of that tension which results from unpleasant states of mind. Laughter contributes distinctly to the production of a more cheerful attitude of mind, and thus fosters endocrine balance. If laughter produces even the slighest effect in the direction of endocrine stimulation, as seems almost inevitable from the conditions, then it means very much for the restoration of endocrine balance. These ductless glands are all affected by each other's secretions, so that whatever the vibratory massage set up by laughter may accomplish, it is sure to affect the whole chain of glands.

CHAPTER VII

LAUGHTER AND THE STOMACH

O F the organs in the abdomen probably the
stomach is more directly affected by laughter, and especially hearty laughter, than any other.
This is due to the mechanical arrangement which
makes the relations between the diaphragm and the
stomach very intimate. The esophagus, or swallowing tube, just before it enters the stomach in its
course from the pharynx, or back of the throat,
passes out of the chest through an opening in the
diaphragm, which for that reason is called the
esophageal opening. This surrounds the lower end
of the swallowing tube very much as a ring fits
on a finger. As the diaphragm moves up and down
in laughter, this opening presses down on the
stomach, and then is lifted upward, and, because
of their intimate connection, agitates the stomach
very freely.

This action of the diaphragm on the stomach is
so direct in its churning effect that it might possibly

be expected to interfere somewhat with the stomach's function. That would probably be true if the stomach's principal function was what it used to be considered to be, the manufacture of digestive secretions. As a matter of fact however stomach secretion is of comparatively little significance for digestion. The rôle of the stomach as a digestive organ was greatly exaggerated in physiology, and above all in pathology, until comparatively recent research cleared up the subject. As a matter of fact the stomach is ever so much less important than it used to be considered, and represents scarcely more than an enlarged end of the swallowing tube, the main purpose of which is not to digest food, but to provide a reservoir or storage place for food so that we may not have to eat more than two or three times a day, and yet have a constant supply of energy-producing material being absorbed for vitality purposes. The best proof of the truth of this lies in the fact that the whole stomach has been removed in certain cases, and the patients have gained in weight and improved very much in health, especially so far as digestion was concerned. In cases where there has been serious interference with stomach motility by the contraction of an ulcer or by some other disturbance of gastric peristalsis, the stomach, by the operation of jejunostomy, is practically made a continuance of the swallowing tube, and scarcely more.

Some thirty years ago, when Schlatter removed nearly the whole stomach, fastening the end of the swallowing tube to the remnant of the stomach that was left, his patient proceeded to gain some forty pounds in weight in the course of the next six months, though eventually, I believe, she died from recurrence elsewhere of the cancer which necessitated the operation upon the stomach. This patient had to be fed liquid food every hour or so during the day but her digestion and assimilation were excellent, though she had no important remnant of her stomach left.

After all, as we have said, the modern operation of jejunostomy—that is, the fastening of a loop of the jejunum, or upper portion of the small intestine, to the stomach so that the stomach may empty itself without having to pass the food through the pylorus or ordinary gateway of the stomach, because there is a stricture or scar there interfering with stomach evacuation—almost completely accomplishes the purpose of eliminating the stomach as an organ of digestion, and leaves it, at most, as only an imperfect sort of storage tank at the end of the swallowing tube.

Stomach secretion is entirely of minor importance and, in a certain number of patients, quite by accident, it has been found that there was no stomach secretion, that is to say, in these patients the food remained unchanged in the stomach for whatever length of time it stayed there. The condition is known as *achylia gastrica*, that is, failure of the stomach to manufacture chyle. The power to modify food in such a way that it will be more or less ready for further digestive processes in the intestines is absent, perhaps by congenital defect. Patients who were the subjects of this affection and who, according to the old idea of dyspepsia, ought to be seriously ill because their stomachs were not capable of digesting, often had complained of no digestive symptoms of any kind, nor exhibited any bad effects, and their curious pathological condition was discovered in some routine examination.

By far the most important function of the stomach is its motor function. We will pardon it for not secreting if it will only pass on the food regularly to the intestine, for the intestines repre-

sent the real place where the digestive processes
are accomplished. This is only what might be expected naturally, seeing that such extremely important secretory organs as the liver and the
pancreas empty their secretions into the intestine,
and that the small intestines themselves are well
above twenty feet long, and, with their folds of
mucous membrane, present a very large surface
for digestive and absorptive purposes. These folds
increase the secretory and absorption mucous membranes by a score of times.

The movements of the diaphragm in laughing
might have interfered with the stomach secretion
and with the intricate and essential peptic processes
which were supposed to occur in the stomach by
preceding generations, but they actually help the
stomach in the motor processes which we have now
come to know are such an important feature of the
stomach's work. For the peristaltic waves, which
go through the stomach as well as the intestines
themselves, cause the stomach to set up a churning
movement in the midst of which a definite selection
of foodstuffs is made so that they may be passed
on in regular order to the intestines.

The stomach's relation to digestion is much more

psychological than physiological in the ordinary sense of those terms. The stomach picks out first the sugars and starches, and then the vegetable proteids, and then the meat proteids, and then the fats, and passes each of these varied foodstuffs on in this order to the intestines for complete and definitive digestion. Just how the stomach is capable of recognizing and picking out from the mass and mess it contains these various food materials, especially in the heterogeneous mixture to be found in the stomach after a heavy meal which consisted of a large variety of materials from fruit cocktail and soup to nuts and cheese, would be very difficult indeed to explain. The physiological chemist, even when most expert, would probably object to being given so intricate a problem as that to solve. Especially the chemist would not take kindly to the task of doing this in the course of a few hours, and in such a confined space as the stomach.

We have given up the idea of the digestive stomach function to a great extent, but the stomach remains a very wonderful organ. We admire it now, however, for something very different from what we thought it was before. During the churning process, as it goes on, the various materials are segregated from each other and passed on to the intestines. Anything that encourages this churning process is sure to do good, and laughter, by the stimulation which it sets up when the ring of the diaphragm crowds down on the cardiac end of the stomach, evidently produces an excellent effect. We all know that laughing during and after meals is an eminently useful adjuvant for digestion, and that the state of mind which goes with laughing is an eminently important factor in making the digestive process more effective than it would otherwise be. Laughter at meals and just after is one of the best aids to stomach disposal of food that we have.

Careful investigation made with the X rays has shown that in animals the emotions which are at the opposite pole from laughter in human beings, fear and panic and anger and hate, stop the digestive process. It has been found, for instance, that in cats, if the cat is fed something that it likes very much with some mixture of materials that are opaque to the X rays, the process of churning these materials in the stomach will go on very happily and successfully while the animal is left to itself. If anything happens, however, to make the animal excited or angry, then the churning process, which represents the peristaltic stomach waves, stops at once, and digestion is manifestly interfered with.

I have seen a laboratory cat which was a general favorite and treated so well by every one that it was sleek and fat and haughty, tried out in this way with very striking results. The laboratory cat is needed to protect caged animals from mice and rats, so there was a very definite regulation that it must not be experimented on, but it was felt that for this once experiments might be made. Some fish that the cat liked very much was bought, and, after a mixture of sufficient bismuth to ensure a shadow with the X rays, the fish in the form the animal liked it best was fed to the cat. The meal was evidently enjoyed very much. The cat purred and expressed its delight at the treatment in very best cat's fashion. It lay sleek and peaceful in the sun. Then its paw was pressed upon by wooden pincers until the cat resented it. The pressure was maintained in spite of the cat's efforts to free itself, though the animal was not injured in any way. After a time it became so angered that it arched its back and spit at its tormenter. It was very interesting to note what happened in the cat's interior.

Peristalsis, with wavelike motion after wavelike motion, had been proceeding very regularly while the cat was in peace, but a few minutes later, when the cat became thoroughly angry, all of this stopped. It was not resumed immediately when the cat was left to itself and its digestion once more. It was actually ten minutes or more before regular stomach peristalsis was resumed again.

Almost needless to say, the cat, in spite of the claims made for it by some fond mistresses of favorite tabbies, has not a very high place in nature, so far as psyche is concerned, and is not considered to be of a lofty degree of intelligence. However low that may be, nevertheless, when you disturb the cat's state of mind in any way its stomach is at once inhibited in its occupation of passing on the various foodstuffs. It is easy to understand that from this stasis to reverse peristalsis, with actual vomiting of the material that had been eaten with so much relish, might readily occur in animals whose intelligence was of a higher order, or in men where the psyche preponderates.

This should be a lesson for those who think that they can save time by reading their mail at table. An Irish physician who had a very lively sense of humor even in his professional work used to say, "Every minute saved from your meals is a dollar in your doctor's pocket a little later on in life." In the full tide of digestion men read letters or telegrams that are very disturbing, and then they wonder why digestion does not proceed normally. The reason is that the disturbance of mind has interfered with the stomach motility, and whenever it is extreme it may even stop peristalsis entirely, and that practically means the end of stomach digestion for some time. The cat's psyche does not continue its hampering of stomach functions for longer than a few minutes, but the emotions of human beings are not so passing in their character, and therefore the disturbance continues sometimes for an hour or more, and sometimes for several hours. No wonder that such people have stomach symptoms. That accounts for the neurotic or psychoneurotic indigestion that is so common at the present time.

We all know, or at least have experienced if we have not noticed it much, a certain contraction in the region of the stomach that takes place whenever we are angered or grieved or depressed. A man may go to table with a fine appetite and be given some bad news that will make it almost impossible for him to eat. It takes his appetite away completely. On the other hand, if he has just eaten heartily before the bad news comes, he will note a disturbance of the stomach area with a sense of tightening about it. This probably represents exactly the sort of thing that was observed in the cat when it was made angry immediately after eating a meal that it liked, and when the peristaltic movement, which was proceeding so regularly and satisfactorily before, stopped completely.

It is easy to understand how the relaxation of this tight feeling or contraction will come as the result of laughter. It actually shakes the stomach, and pushes it down, and allows it to come back as the diaphragm makes its excursions. This agitation of the stomach overcomes the tension in it set up by the feelings which have caused regular peristaltic movements to cease. Nature tempts us to laugh after meals, but, as is so often the case, that temptation is connected with a real benefit to our system and accomplishes a very definite beneficial purpose.

Other elements may interfere with peristalsis and cause digestive symptoms, or at least disarrange it. Coffee, for instance, probably interferes with peristalsis to a certain degree in most people, and that is one of the reasons why it is often not advisable for them to take coffee with their meals or just afterwards. Of course, there are some people who enjoy coffee after meals, and when one of these, a Frenchman, was told that coffee slowed digestion, his reply was, "That must be what I want done with my digestion, my coffee tastes so good to me." Sometimes it is not a bad idea to have digestion proceed a little more slowly, especially if a man has an hour or two of leisure after his meal in which to digest it calmly and quietly. Coffee will tend to keep most people awake, and that is beneficial. Sleep after eating leaves a bad taste in the mouth. The tendency of a full stomach is to induce sleep. Coffee then enables a man to enjoy the satisfaction of the sense of repletion that comes with a good hearty meal. Nothing gives a happier feeling. If, at the same time there is laughter, then digestion becomes one of the joys of life. The slower it proceeds the better, though laughter stimulates the stomach just enough to keep it at its work and enable it to accomplish its pur- pose of gradually passing the load of the stomach on to the intestines, where it more properly belongs, and where there is so much more room for it in the twenty feet and more of small intestines.

How much the effect on the stomach of this up and down movement of the diaphragm in laughter may be, is made clear from the fact that even the chemical secretion of the stomach, such as it is, is produced by a nervous reflex which must take place through the intrinsic ganglion cells of the stomach itself, since the secretions occur even after complete severance of the extrinsic nervous connections with the stomach. The rubbing movement consequent upon laughter that is produced upon the stomach walls must inevitably affect these ganglionic centers. The human stomach, unlike that of the birds, has very thin walls, so that none of the tissue elements in it would be protected from up and down movements of the diaphragm more than by a very thin covering. All our knowledge of the stomach, in a word, tends to make us feel that moderate movements of it, instead of in any way doing harm do good for the processes of digestion. There are old customs among the religious orders especially, involving walking quietly after meals, which point very clearly to the fact that their observation of their members over long periods had shown them that quiet movement after meals was rather good for people. The instinct of young folks which makes them dance at such times is very probably not so deleterious to health as many people claim, and may even be beneficial.

When patients complain of indigestion then it is extremely important to find out not only what is eaten at meals and how much, but also the social conditions under which the eating is done. If the so-called dyspeptic is accustomed to take his meals alone, or perhaps if he eats with others, but occupies himself with his mail, or with the morning newspaper, it is easy to understand that he is predisposing himself to digestive trouble. Meals ought to be taken in cheerful surroundings, and above all with jolly companionship, just as far as possible. There should always be laughter during meals and during the time immediately succeeding the meal. Nature predisposes to it in every way. To neglect the call is surely to suffer for it.

It is not always easy to secure these conditions in ordinary family life, but extremely difficult if the patients are unmarried and have no one with whom they usually take their meals. In family life, unfortunately, meal times are not always looked on as times of jollity, but they ought to be, and the deliberate effort should be made to introduce as much cheer as possible into them. One of the old jokes on marriage is "that married folk do not live longer, but it seems longer." As a matter of fact, however, recently collected statistics have made it very clear that married folks do live longer than the unmarried. I believe that the average length of life of a married man is nearly five years longer than that of his unmarried brother. The bride has a perfect right to say to the groom on the wedding day, "Now I've added five years of expectancy to your life, so take care of it."

It has been suggested that one of the principal factors in this lengthening of life for married folk is that their meals are not taken alone and are usually taken under rather cheery conditions and with an interchange of comment on the news of the day and the little failings of their friends, which usually produces some hearty laughter, or at least some pleasant smiling during the course of the meal. Unmarried folk are much more likely to be solitary, and therefore to miss the beneficial effects of the laughter and cheeriness. Besides, the married folk are more likely to live socially, that is, in contact with others, in such a way that there is at least a pretense of jollity during meals when company is present, or when they are guests of friends. Even though it should be only a pretense, if it involves laughter, that is quite sufficient to stimulate digestion and aid in the alleviation of dyspeptic tendencies so prone to develop where meals are taken alone and there are no jerky diaphragmatic movements to set the stomach actively into peristalsis, and increase secretion.

CHAPTER VIII

LAUGHTER AND THE INTESTINES

IF the long promised visitor from Mars should come down to earth in our day, and should read the medical advertisements in our papers and magazines, he would very probably be inclined to think that intestinal function had broken down among the earth dwellers since so many advertisements proclaim the fact that all sorts of aids for intestinal function are for sale. It is sometimes said that at least five times as much money must be spent in buying materials that are advertised as is spent by the advertiser. Assuming that to be true, it is very probable that many millions of money are expended every year, indeed, there are those who say that it must be hundreds of millions, in remedies that will facilitate intestinal evacuation.

Even with all that supplementary stimulation of intestinal function, there are many physicians who are inclined to say that some of the most serious chronic ailments of mankind are due to inefficient intestinal peristalsis and insufficient evacuation, as the result of which various toxic materials are absorbed from the intestinal tract into the body, with very unfortunate results.

This is not a new development in the history of mankind, for some of us recall what happened, or at least certain remarks that were made, when Matthew Arnold visited this country about fifty years ago. The distinguished English *littérateur*, "the apostle of anti-Pharisaism," as he was called, declared that what we needed, above all, in this country was "sweetness and light." A distinguished New York editor, very well known for his caustic wit and his readiness in making phrases, declared that, if our English visitor would only read the newspapers and magazines, he would find that, while his opinion was that we needed sweetness and light, that of a great many people who were willing to pay to have their advice get to the public, rather than be paid for giving it, was that what we really needed was laxatives and more laxatives. The advertising of such materials was comparatively light in those days to what it has become in our time, but already there was a very noticeable tendency to create in people's minds a feeling that, as a nation, our intestinal function was not at all what it should be, and that it needed jacking up in many ways if we were really to enjoy good health.

All over the world there is a rather definite feeling that the stimulation of intestinal function is extremely important for health. There is at least one distinguished surgeon, and a number of distinguished neurologists, to say nothing of medical clinicians, who are quite convinced that the greater part of the ills of mankind come from sluggishness of their intestines with consequent delay of excrementitious materials and a definite tendency to have absorption of toxic substances as a consequence of that delay. Some of these members of the medical profession have even gone so far as to say that the large intestine is not only the breeder of disease because of absorption of toxic materials from it, but it is actually the great shortener of life.

They are very much inclined to think that nature is in process of eliminating the large intestine as a step in the higher evolution of man, and that the surgeons could do nothing better than to remove it in many cases, so as to help in that process of evolution. This opinion is not shared by many physicians, but it helps to make one understand how important for health the large intestine and its function have now come to be considered. Nothing is more likely to do harm than inefficiency of the intestinal tract, both from the point of view of absorption of food materials and the possibility of the absorption of toxic substances, which may produce rather serious pathological conditions in various delicate structures throughout the body, including the joints, and the heart, and certain of the serous membranes.

Physicians have been very much occupied with the thought of helping intestinal movement, but, of course, have come to realize that the use of medicaments in order to stimulate intestinal function is likely to be followed by unfortunate consequences. Whenever any organic structure in the body has to be stimulated regularly to do its work it loses the habit of function for itself and, after a time, more and more of the stimulant is required to help it to do its work. After a time the organs also become habituated to the stimulation, and will refuse to act unless by ever increased dosing of them. Drug medication for the purpose of bringing about intestinal movements may be of service for a short interval until regularity of evacuation is secured, but to continue it with the idea that it will persist in its effectiveness is a mistake.

Modern physicians therefore have above all tried to secure mechanical methods of encouraging peristalsis, and thus securing proper intestinal function. The Germans were particularly ingenious in the invention of suggestions for this purpose. For instance, a generation ago it was suggested that there should be massage of the abdominal area following the line of the ascending colon and the transverse and then the descending colon so as to encourage intestinal evacuation. This required the services of a trained masseur or masseuse, and therefore could be had at most as only a transient remedial measure. It was next suggested that a sixteen pound round shot could be used by these individual patients and being placed upon the abdomen in the region of the cæcum, the right lower quadrant of the abdomen, might be rolled upward following the course of the colon, and then across and down, following the transverse and descending colon. It should then be lifted over to the other side and the process repeated. In cold weather, however, it was found that a metal ball was extremely uncomfortable and chilling to the patient, and that it even tended to set up a tendency to spasm, which interfered with the intestinal activity. It was then suggested that a heavy bowling ball made of wood, and therefore not so naturally chilly to the touch, because wood does not carry off heat so rapidly as metal, would serve the purpose. A number of people actually used this to advantage. They found, however, that when they were away from home it was rather a difficult matter to carry the ball with them, or to secure another to replace it, so that only those who lived rather fixed lives at home were quite satisfied with this mode of treatment, though it was often very effective.

There is no need, however, for this artificial mechanical massage, for laughter constitutes an excellent method of massaging the large intestine without the necessity for any apparatus, or any auxiliaries. It must be hearty laughter and not merely a little ripple, but there is no need of the exaggerated horse laughter that some people indulge in. In hearty laughter, as we have said, the diaphragm goes up and down five or six inches, thus massaging all the organs above and below it. Ordinarily the intestines are thought of as so low in the abdomen as not to be affected very much by movements of the diaphragm. It must not be forgotten, however, that the large intestine, especially in its transverse portion, which runs across the abdomen just about the level of the navel, is rather close to the diaphragm, and is surely affected by it whenever the laughter is accompanied by anything like full excursions of the diaphragm. It is this portion of the intestines particularly that needs to be stimulated. Running across the abdomen as it does, there is a definite tendency for it to sag in the middle, and this is particularly likely to happen whenever any sluggishness of the intestinal tract is present. As is well known, it is almost impossible, if any weight at all is placed upon a string stretched from one point to another, to keep it from sagging. The transverse colon is in that situation. It is fastened rather firmly at the hepatic flexure, and also at the splenic flexure, but there is a chance for it to sag in between these points. It always does so to some extent, and therefore needs encouragement and stimulation to enable it to continue its peristaltic movements and bring about motion in the intestinal contents. It can be stimulated by means of laughter more simply and surely than in any other way.

Laughter above all encourages peristalsis and stimulates the motor function. Physicians used to be very much occupied with the idea that the main function of the gastrointestinal tract was secretion, but now they know that the motor function is at least as important as the secretory, and that for the beginning of the gastrointestinal tract in the stomach, and for the end of it in the large intestines, motion and the motor function are more important than anything else. Every advance in knowledge with regard to the gastrointestinal tract in recent years has emphasized the importance of the motor function. Laughter which encourages and stimulates motility can readily be understood, then, to be of very great significance for the maintenance of health. For sedentary people particularly laughter is one of the most important modes of exercise of abdominal muscles that humanity has, and the fact that men alone, and not animals, are gifted with it emphasizes its significance.

The movements of the large intestine have in

recent years been found to be much more complex than they were originally considered to be. Cannon of Harvard, from his studies of the normal colonic movements in cats as seen by the Roentgen rays, has reached the conclusion that the movements in the proximal portion of the large intestine are in reverse direction. He divides the large intestine into two parts. These consist of the cæcum and ascending colon as the first part, and the transverse and descending colon as the second part. In the ascending colon and the cæcum, the most frequent movement observed is that of antiperistalsis, that is to say, the bowel churns the food in the direction of the opening from the small intestine, though the presence of the iliocæcal valve prevents the material from passing out of the large intestine. This delay furnishes opportunities for the absorption of fluid, so that the intestinal contents may easily be controlled, but also for the absorption of nutritional material from the intestinal contents before they pass on for evacuation. The second part of the large intestine has its peristalsis in the other direction, but by this time the absorption of fluid leaves the contents of rather solid consistency.

The division between the two parts of the large intestine with their contrary movements occurs about the middle of the transverse colon. This, in normal individuals, would not be far from the umbilicus, or navel. It is easy to understand then, that movements of the diaphragm up and down, the direct effect of which is particularly felt at this point—as can be readily demonstrated by deep inspiration, or in singing, or in laughter—would particularly affect this part of the anatomy and its physiology. Anything that will stimulate the function of the large intestine is extremely important in our time, for constipation is one of the prominent features of life in our day. As was said, millions of dollars are spent every year on laxatives. It would be much more satisfactory and much more wholesome to have the function of the large intestines accomplish itself without artificial stimulation. Laughter however is not artificial, but represents one of the most natural reactions that men and women have, and it has its effect most completely and directly just at the point where there is a division between the two parts of the large intestine for the accomplishment of its purposes.

Besides the large intestine, however, the small intestine also is affected by laughter. Most people are inclined to think of the abdominal cavity as having spaces in it surrounding the various organs. As a matter of fact, there are no empty spaces, and organs rest upon one another, and therefore, any movement which occurs, especially if it is at all extensive, affects all of them. In the abdominal cavity the liver and pancreas and spleen, as well as the kidneys, which are situated at the back and outside of the formal peritoneal cavity, have no free spaces round them, but are directly in contact through peritoneal folds with coils of intestine which have no empty spaces in them, for just as soon as there is no food material present the intestinal mucous membranes fall into contact with each other. This is true also with regard to the stomach. When we feel very "empty" we use a familiar expression for hunger that does not mean that there is a distended stomach gaping for food materials to be poured into it. The stomach distends only in proportion as the food goes into it, and some stomachs have a tendency to contract after a certain amount of food reaches them, so that people who really need to eat more often say that they "feel full," though they may have taken only a comparatively small quantity of food. Their stomachs really are contracted, but what they need is to put more food into them and overcome a certain habit of contraction that has formed, and then there will be no trouble about taking sufficient food.

When the diaphragm moves up and down freely in the midst of all these abdominal organs, pressing them together in intimate contact, all of them are massaged. As the diaphragm moves down, the large muscles that form the abdomen move outward so as to give more room to the organs within the abdominal cavity, and then, as the diaphragm goes up, the abdominal muscles contract so that there may be no vacuum produced within the abdomen. This exercise of the abdominal muscles is unusual for those who have not been accustomed to laughing, and it is perfectly possible to make oneself sore by laughter, as a great many people have realized, to their pain. These movements of the diaphragm, however, massage vigorously all these organs and act with particular advantage on the intestines. It is very probable that the deliberate indulgence in laughter, good hearty laughter, several times a day, on the part of the inhabitants of this country would do more to lessen the present bill for laxatives that the citizens of the United States pay than anything else that could be thought of.

Unfortunately, there is a definite tendency to a vicious circle of disadvantage to the individual whenever laughter does not take place. Sluggishness of the intestines leads to delay of intestinal contents and consequent absorption of undesirable materials from the intestinal tract. These have a definite tendency to produce a certain amount of organic lethargy, with consequent depression. There is a very old tradition that constipated people are not prone to laugh nearly so much as others. The "constipated owl" is held up as a horrible example. The lack of laughter causes deficiency of the motor function of the intestines, and this brings about what the old classical authors used to call tendencies to melancholia, for which they had themselves purged in the springtime. This vicious circle of unfortunate influences may go on emphasizing itself until the patients become prone to sit around and find it very hard to laugh, or at least to get up anything like a good hearty laugh which would break the tightening vicious circle.

Laughter is the best stimulant for the gastro-intestinal tract that we have, and it is probable that in our erect position we need its action very much. The animal on all fours has all its organs fastened to its backbone, swinging rather freely in its pendent abdomen when it moves, while human organs press down upon each other by gravity, and thus encourage sluggish tendencies. Laughter, by stirring up all the organs, relieves this tendency, and hence it is that man has the instinct for laughter as a compensation for his erect position. Unfortunately, a great many people do not use it to the extent that they ought, and thus lose one very health-giving function that they were meant to exercise.

If absorption of food material from the intestines was merely a question of osmosis, that is, the diffusion of fluids through a membrane, a definitely physical process, or if it were due to inequality of concentration in solutions on the two sides of the membrane, laughing might be expected to interfere with this natural process because of the jolting movements in connection with it, especially when it is hearty. It has been definitely demonstrated, however, by physiological investigation that absorption of food materials as it actually takes place is not governed by these merely physical laws and processes, but depends largely upon the properties of the living membrane itself, which is composed of epithelial cells. It is the life quality in the stomach wall which prevents the gastric juice from digesting the stomach tissues, as would take place if the same tissues were put inside the stomach when dead, for the stomach digests tripe, that is the stomach tissues of animals, very well. So, in the intestine, the living cells have to do with absorption just as they resist digestion, and anything that increases their vitality is good for them. The up and down movement of the diaphragm, because of the massage, increases the blood supply, adds to the vitality, and therefore benefits rather than hinders the digestive processes.

CHAPTER IX

LAUGHTER AND THE MIND

WHILE laughing produces all the beneficial effects on the large organs of the body which have been pointed out in the preceding chapters of this book, an almost more important influence for health remains to be noted in the effect of laughter upon the mind. There is nothing which means so much for the lifting of mental depression —so far as that is not absolutely melancholic, or dependent upon some form of chemical intoxication in the system—as good hearty laughter. As the result of what is called so expressively that down-hearted feeling, pulse and respiration both often become slower than normal. This is practically always true if the depression is at all deep. I have seen neurotically depressed patients come into the office breathing as slowly as 14 or 15 to the minute, with heartbeats down below 60 after they had been sitting down for a time, waiting their turn. This is not surprising when the usual pulse respiration ratio is recalled. I have seen these same patients, at the end of a consultation in which they had been brought to take a less serious view of their case, and made to laugh, even though but a little, go out with supra-normal pulse and respiration.

Men who tell good stories whenever the occasion offers and make it their business to collect them so as to regale others with them are sometimes considered to be more than a little of a bore by many busy men who are much preoccupied with their business; but they are real benefactors of mankind, for they lift up people's hearts, quite literally, by means of their diaphragms and set their circulation and respiration going more rapidly than before. The effect upon the mind of this stimulation produced by laughter is very well understood. Long before the days when salesmanship came to be identified with psychology, and when the salesman was just a hired man, and not a specialist in getting men to sign on the dotted line, there were a great many salesmen who were very successful because they knew human nature very well. They always carried a stock of good stories and knew how to fit them to the characters of the men with whom they talked. If a prospective buyer was also a trustee of the church, he was regaled with a very different set of stories from that used effectively on the man who swore a little, drank a little and rather believed in an occasional vulgar story as a sort of safety valve for feelings. The salesman always knew, however, that once a buyer could be made to laugh, almost inevitably it would be an easy thing to get him to give an order. If he could be brought to laugh heartily he was almost inevitably put into the mood to buy ever so much more readily than would otherwise be the case. Laughter makes one expansive in outlook and is very likely to give the feeling that the future need not be the subject of quite so much solicitude as is usually allowed for it.

The effect of laughter upon the mind not only brings relaxation with it, so far as mental tension is concerned, but makes it also less prone to dreads and less solicitous about the future. This favorable effect on the mind influences various functions of the body and makes them healthier than would otherwise be the case. In recent years we have come to appreciate more properly than before the immense significance of the influence of the mind on the body. People get cured of all sorts of complaints—at least they assure themselves that they have been the victims of rather serious disease—by all sorts of curious remedies which prove, after a while, to be utterly inefficacious as therapeutic agents so far as any physical potency in them is concerned. In spite of this absolute negation of therapeutic value so far as their physical effect is concerned, these remedies and modes of healing apparently work veritable miracles of cure. After men and women, and particularly women, have been around to consult half a dozen thoroughly scientific and successful physicians without being benefited in any way, they are cured by some new-fangled mode of treatment. It would seem as though this must represent some very wonderful therapeutic discovery, only after a while the new remedy drops out of sight, because it proves to be utterly null in its physical efficacy. It is abandoned by all when it ceases to carry with it the strong favorable suggestion which gave it its vogue when it was first announced.

It is amusing to see how trivial were some of the modes of treatment which thus proved capable of curing affections that apparently represented real physical ills. Toy electric apparatus, when electricity was a novelty some two hundred years ago, or pseudo-electricity when something of the wonderful power of electricity began to be understood, made what seemed marvelous cures. Hypnotism, which has proved now, when we know more about it, to be only induced hysteria, promised to be a very valuable therapeutic measure for a while. Now we know that, like the old country doctor who threw his patients into "fits," and then cured the "fits," the only therapeutic efficacy of hypnotism was that it induced another form of hysteria to cure the psychoneurosis, or hysteria, that was already present. The Leyden jar proved marvelously effective two hundred years ago in curing chronic cases, but not more so than the radio apparatus in our time, though neither of them has any therapeutic effect on tissues that any one can demonstrate.

It is clear to a demonstration now after these events that it was all a question of the influence of the mind on the body. Concentration of mind on certain tissues disturbs the function of those tissues, and produces symptoms that seem to be serious. Anything that will relax that concentration of at-

ychosomatic *disorders*

tention, and give a patient new confidence in himself, will bring about a cure. This is the only thing that *will* bring about a cure. The affections that are cured by these remedies that fail are particularly the pains and aches, and the lamenesses and disabilities of various kinds that would seem to be, beyond all doubt, physical, but that prove in so many cases to be amenable to mental treatment, and are thus demonstrated to be mental in origin. As time goes on, when people are better educated, instead of the number of these cures diminishing they multiply, and education is evidently making people ever so much more susceptible to suggestion. People take, particularly, the unfavorable suggestions, and so produce various diseases. A little knowledge is a dangerous thing, and is prone to make people think more about themselves and their ills than they should, and then they get cured by all sorts of funny things.

The reason for this state of affairs is not hard to understand when we know even a little about human nature. Whenever we take ourselves too seriously we are prone to note all of our feelings, and, as a result, we are very likely to think that sensations of various kinds which are merely physiological, or surely scarcely more than normal, represent symptoms of disease. We are so important in our own eyes that anything that happens to us becomes of very great significance. Doctors understand this so well that they know better than to treat themselves, and they even recognize how easy it is for them to exaggerate the significance of symptoms in those who are near and dear to them, and so their families are treated by brother physicians.

Many people are inclined to think that others could not possibly have such feelings as they have without complaining a great deal about them. If they go to a physician under these circumstances, and he tries to reassure them and tells them that there is nothing physical the matter, they are very likely to think that the only reason for his making so little of what is the matter with them is that he wants to keep them from worrying about themselves, or else that he does not know his business well. They know from their feelings that there must be something rather serious the matter with them, and they refuse to be reassured, and try some one else. After a while he does not satisfy any better than his colleague predecessor, and so they are tempted to go on seeing physician after physician, all the while quite confident that they know more about themselves than physicians do, and that if the physicians only understood the case properly they would realize that their patient was the victim of a very serious, but insidious and latent affection that was probably different from anything any one had ever suffered from before.

These are the people who make the lives of the quacks and the charlatans profitable. The quacks do not tell them that there is nothing serious the matter with them, or that they ought to forget their symptoms. On the contrary the quacks are very likely to assure them that they have a very serious affection, and that indeed the reason why other physicians have not recognized the meaning of their symptoms is that, as yet, this particular disease is known only to a very few, one of whom, fortunately for the patients, is the man who is now treating them. He assures them that he understands their cases completely, that he is surprised that they have been able to stand their ills so well, for only a person of very determined will could possibly have borne up under the affliction which they are suffering from, but fortunately he knows how to cure them. It will take some time of course, the process will be somewhat complex, and there may even be setbacks in the healing, but they will surely be cured, though no one else, probably, in the country, could have cured them except the man to whom they have providentially applied. Of course it will cost them a good round sum of money, but then health is a very precious possession, and who will not give up even all that he possesses for health and life?

Thus these serious-minded people get cured. A typical example of the way that they are cured is to be found in the investigation of a cure by radio apparatus in one of our large cities. The healer declared that the vibrations which went through a radio apparatus were quite sure to cure the chronic ills of mankind, for the relief of which all other remedies had failed. The operator proved very successful in healing a number of people. He did not use a battery radio apparatus, but just one of those that works with a crystal. He replaced the ear phones, which are necessary in such an apparatus, by two bunches of mineral wool, the kind that may be bought in the five and ten cent stores. It is used for wiping the rust off iron pots and cleaning kitchenware generally. These bunches of mineral wool were rubbed up and down the affected part of the patient, and it is easy to understand that his feelings told him that something was happening. The operator assured him that his feelings were due to vibrations, which were flowing through him from distant Los Angeles, and from Germany, and from Havana, and Montreal (the vibrations from these two cities seemed to do the men particularly a great deal of good) and then the patient proceeded to get cured. The fee was one hundred dollars a cure, and the operator decided when you had to pay it, and he made a lot of money and had a lot of patients, who sent other patients, until finally a few of them got together and decided that they were not cured. They brought the matter to the police.

One of these healing radio apparatuses was investigated by experts from the police department, and the wires were found to be wrongly connected, so that it would have been impossible to hear a clap of thunder a mile away over it. No vibrations of any kind were going through it, but a lot of people were cured by it, and they were willing to pay a hundred dollars for the cure, and it was "cured" patients who sent many other patients, so that the radio apparatus healer had a crowd coming to him regularly and was making a great deal of money. He was curing people of all sorts of pains and aches and lameness—lame backs and lame shoulders, lame arms and lame wrists, lame ankles and lame legs, lumbago and sciatica, and all sorts of neuritis and neuroses, but then these are the standard set of diseases that get cured by all the new-fangled remedies which prove, after a while, to do no good. When one of his students said to Trousseau, the great French professor of medicine, "They tell me I have consumption, do you think I ought to use that new remedy that is said to be curing so many consumptives?" the great physician said, "Oh, yes, and take it now while it cures, because after a while they will find that it doesn't cure, and then it will not do you any good." How many such "cures" there have been since!

Coué sized up the situation in the modern time very well when he proceeded to tell people to say to themselves, every morning when they awoke, "Every day, in every way, I am getting better and better." If only he had properly diagnosed his cases and eliminated those which had physical disease, he would have been a great benefactor to mankind. I had the privilege of meeting him several times, and of course, as every one knows, he used to say, "I never cure any one, I merely show them how to cure themselves." And this was exactly what he could do for most of the patients who came to him, for they were people who, by taking themselves too seriously, and thinking about their feelings, and dwelling on their sensations, had become persuaded that they were ill, and then were saying to themselves every morning when they awoke—and a great many other times during the day, "Every day, in every way, I am getting worse and worse," very often adding, "I suppose it will not be long before I shall be crippled and unable to do anything, or shall be suffering from some complication of my affection that will carry me off." For people are prone to be pessimistic and to make the worst of things, and if Coué had done nothing else except make them optimistic, that would have meant a very great deal for the betterment of most of them.

Altogether some twenty thousand people went to Coué every year, and, according to the reports that we have, two-thirds of them were cured, and nearly one-half of the remainder were somewhat benefited, leaving only about one in six who felt that they had not been helped by his ministrations. His method seems entirely too superficial to mean anything for the ailments of humanity, and yet the results speak for themselves. Of course it is perfectly clear now that all those who were cured by Coué had nothing physical the matter with them, except, perhaps, certain physical symptoms consequent upon neglect of eating, air, and exercise, which had developed as a result of the persuasion that they were ill, and therefore must limit their diet and exertion, as well as the conviction that they needed so much rest that they did not get out into the air enough. Apart from these factitious elements, superadded to their feelings because of their mental state, these patients were well, only they needed the courage to face life and its trials without giving way under them. When they gave way they lost control of their nerves in various ways, and as a result suffered from what the physicians have come to call psychoneuroses, which is only a nice long Greek name for what used to be called hysteria. Hysteria is only supersuggestibility, that is, too great a tendency to take suggestions and particularly to take unfavorable suggestions.

Coué substituted favorable suggestions for unfavorable ones, and had people keep repeating them until they found an entrance into the mind; then they were better at once and proceeded to get well entirely. To be able to laugh at many of the dreads and fears of life, or at least to laugh at the humorous things, even though these dreads and fears may be disturbing us, is the best possible antidote for the hysterical conditions. Hysterical people take themselves too seriously. They like to attract attention. They like to be in the limelight. If they are suffering from some condition that the ordinary physicians do not seem able to cure, that is a source of great satisfaction to them. To be the victim of some affection that the doctors cannot quite understand, and that ordinary remedies do not avail to relieve, that represents a consummation devoutly to be wished by the psychoneurotic. They like to talk about themselves and their ills, and whenever they do so they make further unfavorable suggestions to themselves, until, finally, they are in a condition where life has become almost intolerable, they are so constantly solicitous lest something serious should happen to them, though, often, after years of complaining, they are willing to confess that nothing of any moment has ever happened.

The only trouble with Coué's system was that there was no proper differential diagnosis of the patients whom he treated. He was not a physician himself—he had been a druggist for a while—he knew nothing about pathology, and even less, if possible, about the niceties of modern diagnostic developments. As a result of this, though by natural selection only the neurotic patients came to him, to a great extent, about one in six of the patients who came to him were not only not benefited, but the delay in applying proper remedies and modes of treatment to them usually made their conditions worse than before, and had a tendency to sink them into depression with regard to themselves. This made it extremely difficult for them to call upon their resources of reactive vitality to help them to get over the physical conditions from which they were suffering when proper remedies were applied. It is easy to understand that cancer cases would be seriously hurt by the delay in seeking proper surgical treatment, diabetic cases injured by neglect of proper diet, and tuberculosis cases that had any active growth of the tubercle bacilli, distinctly set back for lack of rest. It is probable even, that heart and kidney cases would be injured in the same way.

A happy state of mind, such as is induced by favorable suggestion of the Coué order, or by simple laughter, may help in the treatment of these organic diseases, but only after there has been a definite institution of such physical treatment as will correct the natural course of the disease to get worse.

How often do we not hear the expression, "Isn't it wonderful the influence that the mind has on the body, for the cure of disease?" The first part of this proposition is absolutely correct. The mind has a wonderful influence on the body, but the second part of it is wrong entirely, unless the kind of disease that the mind cures is pointed out. What the mind does to the body is that it produces symptoms in it. It can produce the symptoms of any disease. Mental solicitude has been known to produce a simulation of a tumor in certain regions of the body, apparently by the production of a spasm of muscles. The mind has been known to stop menstruation and produce all the symptoms of pregnancy, though after a while there proved to be no physical basis for the symptoms. Queens who married late in life, and greatly wanted an heir for the dynasty, have so worked upon their genital systems that they have produced the symptoms of pregnancy to such an extent as even to deceive skilled attending physicians. Young women who have been indiscreet sexually, and fear intensely the results of their indiscretion, have caused inhibitions of function that seemed to have similar indications, though subsequent developments proved there was nothing significant in them.

The mind can produce symptoms in every organ of the body. It can bring on feelings of depression in the heart which we describe as disheartenment or discouragement, and there will be actual slowing of the pulse and reduction of blood pressure as a consequence. It will rather seriously affect the stomach with the production of nausea and vomiting. Ship doctors will tell you that a good deal more than half the seasickness that occurs in trips across the Atlantic is really due to the mental persuasion of women, and even not a few men, that they are going to be sick, and then they proceed to suffer from it. The same thing is true for a great many other functions, including even that presumedly very physical one of peristaltic movement of the intestines. This is very largely under the influence of habit and the mental state, and it is extremely important to remember this in our day, when so many people are taking remedies of various kinds to encourage peristalsis. Often all they need is a free state of mind with regard to their intestinal functions, and some good hearty laughter to encourage peristalsis, and they would not need to take medicine. This may seem an optimistic point of view and perhaps be considered not justified by actual results, but any physician who has had to treat nervous patients for a number of years will realize at once how much of truth there is in it. Overattention is inhibitory, wholesome neglect and leaving to nature is good therapy, and laughter will add the stimulant element toward convalescence that is so often needed.

In a word the state of mind that is induced by hearty laughter is an excellent therapeutic element because it keeps the mind from inhibiting bodily function. There is an old proverb that a watched pot does not boil, meaning that if you are watching and waiting for water to boil it seems a dreadfully long time. Something of this same thing is true with regard to the watching of any of the functions of the body, and one of the most important therapeutic pieces of advice is to forget about them and go on with the natural course of things. There is nothing that makes us forget so completely about functions of the body that we may have been solicitous over as good hearty laughter. It dissipates the intense concentration of attention on some bodily function, which so often proves to be the principal cause of the disturbance in that function. All the varied "cures" that have cured for a while, and then would not cure anything, demonstrate that the state of mind is the most important thing in the world for a great many patients.

It is no use telling these patients, as a rule, to forget their ills, because usually they have nothing else much to occupy themselves with, and the mind cannot be a blank, but must have something to occupy it. Tell them to laugh, not at themselves, though after a while they will realize that they have been eminently laughable, but to laugh at anything else that can possibly raise a smile. If they could be brought to take the laugh cure a great many of them would proceed to get better at once. They are taking their feelings too seriously. Sometimes the development of a serious interest in anything else will cure them. I have known a man to get over nervous indigestion when his only child suffered from pneumonia. I have known a doctor to forget a whole series of symptoms that he was fostering, when his boy was in the war and he was worried about him. David Harum said, "It's a mighty good thing for a dog to have fleas, because it keeps him from thinking too much about the fact that he's a dog." Diversion of mind is the most important thing in the world. Laughter constitutes the best diversion that we have. The laugh cure will beat all the new-fangled methods of healing, if we can only get people to take it with confidence.

CHAPTER X

LAUGHTER AND SURGERY

ORDINARILY the presumption would be that laughter has no place in association with surgery. The direct physical effect of laughter is to produce a certain amount of quaking of tissues, with vibrations that extend far beyond the region of the diaphragm, which is primarily involved. After surgical intervention rest is a positive indication, as a rule, so that tissues may agglutinate without disturbance of any kind, and so that the adhesion of cut surfaces may be accomplished without any delay or interference. The more serious the operation, and, of course, the nearer it is to the group of organs that are particularly affected by the up and down excursions of the diaphragm, the more necessity there is for absolute quiet of the tissues, and rest must be the watchword. There is no doubt at all that close to important operations, either in time or tissue, laughing must not be indulged in, and of course, above all, must not be encouraged in any way. Surgeons usually make provision that there will not be any disturbance of tissues by prescribing opiates to have their effect during the first few days.

After all, however, this represents only a very small part of the time that the patient has to be under the care of the surgeon and his assistants. Besides the three or four days, or even the week, that may be necessary in order to secure union by first intention, or the nearest to that that may be hoped for, the patient's convalescence may occupy two or three weeks, or even a month or more, and during this time the patient's state of mind is extremely important, not only for his general health, but particularly for the increase of natural vitality that will make the necessary repair of tissues as complete and as thorough as possible.

In the chronic cases, where sometimes the patient will be in the hospital in preparation for the operation for a week or more, his state of mind is also important, and, facing an operation, he must be put in as cheerful a mental condition as can be secured. It is under these circumstances that laughter finds a distinct place in the practice of the surgeon. No one knows better than the experienced surgeon the necessity for cheerfulness, and good hearty laughter is an important factor for this. After all, the patient's ordinary functions must go on as perfectly as possible, both during the time of preparation for an operation, and in the stage of convalescence after the acute conditions immediately following the operation have subsided. This healthy functioning is a consummation devoutly to be wished, and it is helped along by the exercise and massage of organs that come with laughter better than any other way, especially while the patient is confined to bed.

Surgeons have always recognized this as a rule, and the surprise is how long ago they came to appreciate the significance of it, and how ready they were to suggest very explicitly the necessity for deliberately cultivating the cheery state of mind with accompanying laughter, which we are discussing here. Strange as it may seem, one of the greatest of surgeons of the modern time (extending the word modern to mean anything that is not ancient history), Mondeville, the professor of surgery at the University of Paris toward the end of the thirteenth century, was particularly emphatic on this point. He said, "Let the surgeon take care to regulate the whole regimen of the patient's life for joy and happiness by promising that he will soon be well." This would seem only the vague recognition of the fact that a surgical patient must not be allowed to become moody, and that the surgeon himself must encourage him in every way and keep an atmosphere of hope around him.

Mondeville meant ever so much more than this, however, for he proceeds to say that this atmosphere of joy and happiness will be best secured "by allowing his relatives and special friends to cheer him, and by having some one to tell him jokes." In a word, he recognized very thoroughly the help there might be in laughter, and deliberately planned so that his patient would be sure to exercise the diaphragm and massage the large organs that are in anatomical relations with it, though he himself had sufficiently hazy notions, perhaps, as regards some of these relations, or even the importance of some of the organs. He added, "The surgeon must forbid anger, hatred and sadness in the patient, and remind him that the body grows fat from joy and thin from sadness." Here is probably one of the earliest forms of that expression, "laugh and grow fat," though Mondeville mentions it as if it were a maxim of health that had been known for a long time and had been frequently appealed to by those who wanted to improve the condition of a patient's health—as it undoubtedly was.

Mondeville was a very human as well as humane surgeon. He seems to have been a lover of music, and there is no doubt that he thoroughly appreciated how much music might mean for inducing favorable feelings in the mind of the patient who needed his surgical services. He said, "Let the patient be solaced also [this was just after he had suggested that there should be some one to tell him jokes] by music on the viol or psaltery." I have often wondered why music was not more employed in hospitals. There is only one hospital that I have ever known where they made a special effort to use the influence of music for the cheering of patients as they lay in the wards. This was at St. Mary's, Niagara Falls, where the organ in the chapel, by means of electrical connections, could be heard in the wards. I suppose, however, that at the present time all hospital wards are fitted up with radio apparatus, and that they are receiving the various jazz concerts, though I doubt whether this would quite satisfy Mondeville, or fulfill properly his injunctions that the patients "be solaced also by music on the viol or psaltery."

Mondeville emphasized the fact that he did not like garrulous or talkative attendants on the sick, who liked particularly to narrate their various experiences on serious cases, and had a tendency to tell about unexpected deaths that took place while they were taking care of patients. He did not hesitate to say that sometimes near relatives are particularly likely to disturb patients. "Especially are they prone to let drop some hint of bad news, which the surgeon may have revealed to them in secret, or they may even repeat the reports that they may hear from others, or rumors of various kinds from friends or enemies, and this provokes the patient to anger or anxiety and is likely to give him fever."

This medieval surgeon, who has come to be looked upon as one of the great representative surgeons of all times, objected very much to having solemn, long-faced attendants on the sick, and above all he did not want to hear of grouchiness or murmuring about conditions in the presence of the sick. He said, "All of these things will disturb the patients and produce worry and anxiety or fever." His further direction was, "The surgeon therefore, must be careful in the selection of his nurses, for some of them obey very well while he is present, but do as they like, and often just exactly the opposite of what he has directed, when he is away." Mondeville did not like to have wives nurse their husbands because he feared that they would be too serious and too solicitous, and apparently, also, that their familiarity with their husbands kept them from being a source of cheerfulness. He seems to have had another thought, however, that is very different from modern feelings in the matter. Apparently the thriftiness of some of the French wives of that time led them to be over-economical or even stingy, and therefore not quite as ready to get things that would do their husbands good as they ought to be. Mondeville seems to have been a bachelor himself, as a number of these great surgeon-teachers were, because professors of the universities, as a rule, were not permitted to marry, for monastic influences prevailed.

Perhaps that fact will account for Mondeville's expression. "In our days in this Gallican part of the world, wives rule their husbands, and the men for the most part permit themselves to be ruled. Whatever a surgeon may order for the cure of a husband will sometimes seem to wives to be a waste of good material, though the men seem to be quite willing to get anything that may be ordered for the cure of their wives. The whole cause of this seems to be that every woman seems to think that her husband is not as good as those of other women whom she sees around her." In commenting on this very interesting and, from a social aspect, revelatory paragraph in my volume on *Old Time Makers of Medicine*, from which much of this material is taken, I said that "it would be very interesting to know how Mondeville was brought to a conclusion as regards the mutual estimation of husbands and wives in each other's minds that is so different from modern experience in this matter."

It is perfectly certain, however, that Mondeville believed thoroughly in the therapeutic value of laughter, and had seen its importance exemplified a number of times in his practice. We have his textbook of surgery, though it was not printed until toward the end of the nineteenth century. It is looked upon as a landmark in the history of surgery because it is very clearly made up to a great extent out of Mondeville's own surgical experiences. He knew the books of his predecessors well, and especially that of Lanfranc, the great Italian surgeon who brought the surgery of Italy with him over to Paris. Mondeville represents, indeed, a culmination of the surgical experience of two centuries in two countries.

Mondeville's rule then, that the surgeon must have some one to tell his patients jokes, and that he himself "should comfort his patients by pleasant discourse and should always accede to their requests if these do not interfere with the cure of the disease" would seem to be good surgical procedure full six and a half centuries after he first laid it down. Few men have ever thought more highly of their specialty than Mondeville. He deprecated very much that a series of unworthy men "now proceed to make physicians or surgeons of themselves in order to make their living under the cloak of healing." He was sure that "this, our art of surgery which is the third part of medicine [the other two parts were diet and drugs] is with all due reverence to physicians considered by us surgeons ourselves, and by the non-medical as a more certain, nobler, securer, more perfect, more necessary, more lucrative art than the other parts of medicine." He had more than the usual pride in his specialty though that has always been very noticeable among surgeons.

He said further: "It follows from this that the perfect surgeon is more than the perfect physician and that while he must know medicine, he must, in addition, know his surgical technique." And yet, with all this, he repeats with approval the expression of Avicenna, "Often the confidence of the patient in his physician does more for the cure of his disease than the physician with all his remedies."

Mondeville represents the climax of a great surgical period that came at a time when men were developing every phase of human thought marvelously, for he was the product of the end of that glorious period that has been spoken of as "the thirteenth, greatest of centuries." He formulated the traditions of his time, and it is not until this generation that surgeons have come round to doing better work than he was doing. His opinion, therefore, with regard to laughter in its relation to surgical patients is not only interesting but sug-

gestively valuable at all times. It might possibly
be thought that he represented old-fashioned surgery, so unlike ours that its principles would have
no meaning in our time, but he boasted of getting
union by first intention and manifestly succeeded
in doing excellent surgical work. As a matter of
fact modern surgeons feel very much as he did with
regard to the atmosphere of cheer and jollity that
they would like to have among their surgical patients. This was illustrated very well by the conditions that were fostered and encouraged in every
way among the wounded soldiers during the Great
War. Wards were places not of gloom and of
glumness, but, on the contrary, of light-hearted
jesting and hearty laughter whenever an occasion
could be found or made for it.

The place of laughter in surgery is very well
illustrated by some passages from a series of letters from just behind the front in France, written
by an American girl, and published under the
pseudonym "Mademoiselle Miss." It was the early
months of the War in 1915 and they were very
sadly handicapped in their hospital work by the
lack of proper supplies. She had only one hypo-
dermic needle to give injections to over thirty badly

wounded soldiers, only one thermometer to take their temperatures, and they were sadly lacking in gauze and cotton and nearly every surgical supply that is usually considered indispensable. Many of the men were very badly wounded, some of them were dying from peritonitis, others from tetanus. As the patients got even a little better they were moved farther back behind the lines so as to make room for the urgent cases which needed immediate surgical intervention, that were constantly making demands for beds.

It is easy to understand that under the circumstances life was not a very cheery affair in such a front hospital, but the American nurse had succeeded in making it clean, though only by dint of much strategy. As she says herself, "It used to be awful, but there are two ways of appealing to a Frenchman [and surely to nearly every other man], through his heart and through his pride. When you work both together you have his body and soul. And so when my orderlies saw me on my knees, scrubbing, they came to the rescue, and then I clinched the matter with the suggestion that *ours* should be the model ward. It worked."

She says, with regard to the state of cheerfulness

in the wards: "You can't imagine, I suppose, that we laugh and jest all day long? Yet so it is, and if you can't do that you might as well get out for all the good you will ever do a *French* wounded soldier. Why, I believe his very wounds wouldn't heal if he were not allowed to make merry over them, and even jest with you up to the hour before he dies—a mixture of wit and pathos too poignant ever to reproduce."

She adds farther on, "We ought to be joyous here even if men do try to make it a vale of tears; the more suffering I see the more I think so." She tells of young fellows who joked partly to assuage their own pain and partly "to encourage the others." One day when she was about to pour 95 per cent alcohol into a gaping wound, for antiseptics had to be used that were much more powerful than in ordinary peace surgery, it is easy to understand that there was going to be intense suffering, so she was glad the patient had his little joke at it. She had been made a lieutenant in the French army, and wore her insignia, and it was just as she was about to pour the alcohol that the young fellow took the opportunity to say, "What's your rank, mademoiselle?" "I told him. 'Then

I think they should call you lieutenant of the life guards.'" As the patient gripped the sides of the operating table to keep from upsetting the nurse's paraphernalia in the midst of his writhings from the pain, he said with a quizzical look, "Sister, why are you tempting me so when you know very well the government has strictly forbidden our taking any sort of alcohol?"

The most interesting thing about this experience of the American nurse was that it lifted her out of a state of nervous tension from which she had been suffering for some time. In spite of her fourteen hours of daily labor with the blood and anguish of the hospital, she writes that she "began, for the first time in her life, to feel as a normal being should." Her efforts to keep the patients in her ward cheerful, to think always of them and what she could do for them, to plan what might bring them interest and forgetfulness of their conditions, above all to be in intimate touch with real suffering so that she forgot her own petty annoyances and discouragement, all these served to give her a happier outlook on life than she had had before.

We had in New York, just at the beginning of the twentieth century, an interesting illustration of the value of cheerfulness, fresh air, laughter and the opportunity to play for surgical cases in children that deserves to be recalled. There were in the New York City hospitals a number of children suffering from surgical tuberculosis. All of them had been there for months, some of them for several years, and a few of them for as long as five or six years. As a rule, whenever, in the rotation of services, a surgeon came on duty, he would undertake some surgical intervention that he hoped would help these cases. As the result of the intervention, the little patient would be better after a time, and there would be the hope that a radical cure would be effected, but in most of the cases relapse would take place, tissues would break down again, sinuses would be reëstablished, and the patient would be left until the next change of surgeons brought in a period of renewed interest. They represented a very discouraging group of cases for whom it was felt that modern surgery could afford very little enduring relief.

Shortly before this time New York had established down at Sea Breeze, not far from Coney Island, a series of wooden barracks in which mothers with ailing children who needed fresh air more than anything else in the world were taken care of during the summer months. There had been some very interesting experiences with the cure of surgical tuberculosis along the shores of Normandy, where the coldness of water and air, and the dampness would seem to be rather unfavorable factors for such cases. These experiences set the New York health authorities to thinking that perhaps something might be done during even the colder months of the year for tuberculous children down at Sea Breeze. As a result, many of the chronic cases were transferred down there, though the heating arrangements were very inadequate, and the temperature of the wards was often below fifty, especially as the rule was maintained of keeping the windows open. Nurses, except when actually engaged in surgical duties, went around in hoods and shawls, and visiting physicians and surgeons wore their hats and overcoats. The children played in the sand of the seashore near by, often even in the midst of a snowstorm, but were happy and hearty and cheerful, and, above all, laughed most of the time, for hospital decorum was not insisted on. Occasionally bandages would slip down and sand would get into sinuses, but apparently no harm was done, and it was not long before patients began to improve very much, and the improvement that they secured proved enduring, though before this amelioration had so often been followed by relapse and the breaking down of tissues once more.

Patients who had been for years in all the comfort of a New York City hospital, where the temperature was equable and warm, without much benefit were now greatly and rapidly improved in the conditions at Sea Breeze. A great deal of this was due to the stimulating outdoor air. Still more of it, perhaps, was due to the sunshine in which the children played just as soon as they were allowed, or could steal, the permission. We have come to realize now that the glass in the hospital windows kept from them much of the violet end of the spectrum, which was so important for health and vitality, and above all for the stimulation of recuperative powers. Not a little of the therapeutic effects that were so valuable for them were due, however, to the laughter that was so common among them and that bubbled out on every occasion.

One of the very important improvements that was noted almost at once was that after the first week down at Sea Breeze the "starting pains" which so often disturbed these little patients at night ceased to recur. Just as soon as children are not in pain, then the play instinct bubbles over and they begin to laugh and joke at even the slightest thing. The nurses in their shawls, the doctors in their coats and hats and gloves very often were subjects for merriment. The children themselves had become accustomed to the cold air and just radiated cheerfulness and good fellowship, and laughed and joked and proceeded to get well.

The institutional atmosphere is always rather solemn and is likely to be dominated by older people, and that constitutes very probably the most important reason why children do not get on well in institutions. Children's wards in connection with a general hospital are likely to be rather serious and overshadowing of the childish play spirit. Older patients must have silence in order to be permitted to enjoy their solicitude over themselves. Surcease of pain is the signal for the child to be joyful and laugh heartily if there is any occasion for it, and no real reason is needed. In children's hospitals conditions in that regard are likely to be much better, but even there, in the old days, seriousness was maintained to a degree that surely did harm. Children are perhaps the best illustration of how much laughter may have of beneficial influence in surgical cases. It is among crippled children suffering from serious joint disease that one finds oftener than anywhere else in hospital work "the smile that won't come off." Extremely pitiable little victims of pain and suffering they seem to be, and yet, if you go through the wards when they are asleep, very often you will find smiles on their faces; but always during the day when you go through, if you give them any occasion at all, they will laugh with you and at you. No wonder so many of them get well, in spite of the serious tuberculous bone conditions from which they suffer.

Laughter has a real place in surgery at all times. It stimulates the circulation, massages the large organs and increases their function, produces an additional flow of blood to the ductless glands which empty their secretion directly into the blood stream, and thus increases resistive vitality against microbes. To have the blood flow more freely is almost the equivalent of introducing a fresh supply of blood into the veins, and laughter very probably has an effect distantly resembling blood transfusion. Blood is ever so much better oxidized because of deeper breathing in the midst of laughter, and this is sufficient of itself to make patients less sensitive. It has been noted that if patients are asked to draw a series of deep breaths so that they cause their blood to take up more oxygen than normal, certain brief operations, like the opening of an abscess, or even the pulling of a tooth, may be performed without the infliction of nearly so much pain as would otherwise be the case. Laughter accomplishes something of the same purpose of blood superoxidation.

In a word laughter develops recuperative powers, and it was the observation of this fact that led the medieval surgeons to encourage it so heartily. It acts both on patients' minds and bodies, and predisposes all the natural means of cure to act to the best possible advantage. Surgeons have often remarked that their patients who are in wards, that is, where they are always in company with others, seem as a rule, to get on better, when suffering from similar conditions, than those who are in private rooms. It might seem that the greater care extended to private patients would surely lead to their more rapid convalescence, but it does not. The air of a ward is likely to be much more human, there is sure to be more of laughter in it, and of heartfelt sympathy with others, and therefore less solicitude about self. The fact that other people around are suffering arouses sympathy and leads to self-repression and self-control, but also it fosters efforts to make others round one cheery, and any such effort is sure to be reflected back on one's self and add to one's own good feeling.

All this has been known, but it has not been consciously recognized, nor quite deliberately put into effect. One of the things that a surgeon needs to think of is the provision of such an atmosphere as will surely lead his patients to laugh rather freely and not to take their condition too seriously.

CHAPTER XI

LAUGHING AND OTHER DIAPHRAGM ACTIVITIES

TO understand the place of laughter in the body and its effect upon health, it is absolutely essential to study the other movements of the diaphragm which occur, and which nearly all have very definite purposes for the preservation of health and the defense of the organism against various disturbing agents. The diaphragmatic movements apart from respiration are much more varied than are usually thought, and each one of them has a definite significance. Some of them are very important for health.

PHYSICAL DIAPHRAGM ACTIVITIES

Coughing.—The most familiar one is coughing. This is a sudden reflex spasm of the diaphragm caused by the presence of irritating materials in the larynx, or larger, or even smaller, bronchi and meant to bring about the expulsion of the irritating materials. Almost needless to say, coughing is an extremely important function. When patients are too weak to cough, respiratory disturbances at once become serious, that is, ever so much more serious than they would be if the coughing reaction could be successfully produced. In very young children, that is in infants, their failure to cough makes them ready victims of respiratory ills that a little bit later in life they would be able to throw off very well. Later on in life, when patients are very weak from age, or from debility due to disease, the danger from respiratory affections increases greatly and a great many of the deaths of old age are due to failure on the part of patients to cough up material and help nature to remove not only mucus and other clogging materials, but also microörganisms, whose multiplication adds to the danger of the affection.

There was a time not so long ago when a variety of remedies were prescribed with the idea of lessening cough, but physicians are rather careful now, as a rule, not to interfere with it unless there are very special reasons for doing so. There are times when sleep is so much disturbed by cough, or when a weak patient is being racked very much by it, that a physician may choose between two evils and lessen the cough by opiates. What he much prefers to do, however, is to encourage the cough just as much as possible, so as to relieve the bronchial tissues from the presence of material that is interfering with their function. The mucus, which is thrown out by nature in larger quantities than in health, is meant to carry with it the microbes whose presence has caused the inflammatory reaction in the bronchi that we know as bronchitis. Their removal must be secured and anything that would delay their removal is likely to do ever so much more harm than good. Cough is then a thoroughly conservative reaction on the part of the diaphragm as the result of reflexes from the terminal nerve endings in the bronchioles and the larger bronchi.

Whenever a foreign body finds its way into the larynx, or there is even threat of that, there is a sudden spasm of the diaphragm with strong convulsive coughing which expels the offending material. We all know what a sudden spasm of coughing comes over us when, for instance, in drinking, some drops of fluid find their way "down the wrong way." Of course they do not find their way "down the wrong way" because that would be down the air tubes into the lungs, and any such diversion of food material would surely be fatal. What happens is that a very small quantity finds its way on to the very sensitive tissues in the neighborhood of the larynx, and at once a spasm of coughing brings about such expulsive respiration as removes the particles.

But this is not the whole story of coughing. It is not merely an instinctive or organic reflex. Coughing is, to a considerable extent, under the influence of the mind. It is well known that coughing is contagious. In church in the winter time, if during portions of the services people have been bowing reverently, when the heads go up there will usually be a discreet, modest cough or two somewhere in the church, and then, as if people were reminded of it, a number of coughs, and then, particularly if it is a damp day, a whole battery of coughs is let off in all parts of the church. Public speakers are likely to know that if somebody in the audience is taken with a persistent cough, others are quite sure to follow suit and it will require very special exercise of tactfulness, and perhaps the telling of a good story that will bring a laugh from everybody, before the coughing disturbance will be put an end to. It might seem as though coughing would always be a physical reaction, but it can be due merely to a mental suggestion. This is what must be recalled with regard to all the diaphragm activities.

Sneezing.—There is another spasmodic movement of the diaphragm, very much resembling coughing in many ways, that represents an important protective activity on the part of nature. This is sneezing. It occurs whenever irritant particles enter the nose and lodge on the nasal mucous membrane. Snuff, for instance, occasions it, but so does pepper, and so will ordinary dust. People whose mucous membranes are particularly sensitive suffer from a great deal of sneezing and irritation of the mucous membranes of their throat and nose and eyes as the result of the pollen of certain plants, and particularly certain weeds. These "hay fever" patients, as they are called, may suffer from either spring or fall pollen, or from plain summer dust. Rose cold is very familiar in the spring, and then comes hay fever in the summer, and finally the fall catarrh from the ragweed and other such plants.

In all these patients there is a great deal of

sneezing in order to throw off, if possible, the irritative substances. The mucous membranes of the respiratory tract, however, become congested, there is considerable flow of secretion, and the patients sneeze a great deal without securing much relief until they get away from the irritant material, whatever it may be, or until the change in the season makes the particular plant incapable of producing the irritant material.

Sneezing would seem to be a very definite physical reflex, without any mental element, and without any tendency to contagion. A certain number of cases have been described, however, in which there would seem to be definite mental elements. For instance, a lady who suffered every year from rose cold when the roses appeared was surprised one year before she thought the roses were out at having some one bring a large, full-blown rose into the room. It was not long then before she began to have symptoms of rose cold, and sneezing with it. The rose proved, however, to be artificial, and of course produced no pollen, so that the nasal affection and the sneezing were entirely due to the mental influence. It has often been noted that when hay fever patients congregate in groups there is much more likely to be more sneezing than where they are out of sound of each other. Much slighter irritation is capable of producing sneezing under circumstances where the mind is reminded of it than otherwise. It has even been noted that where hay fever patients talk a good deal about sneezing they sneeze much more frequently than would otherwise be the case. The mental element and a certain psychical contagiousness are connected with it, as with all the diaphragmatic activities.

Animal Emanation Asthma.—It has been suggested that the tendency for some people to have distinct irritation of the respiratory mucous membrane, as the result of intimate association with animals, is a mental rather than physical state. Careful observations that have been made, however, make it very clear that this is a real physical condition. The presence in their sleeping room of a cat which has wandered in from a balcony or fire escape is quite sufficient to wake some people up and make them realize that there is a cat in the room. In the old days when people rode behind horses, a certain small number of them suffered from horse asthma and would have a few sneezes at night before going to bed, and then awake in an asthmatic attack during the night. I have known a patient to suffer from asthma which began with sneezing as the result of sleeping on goose feathers. Other varieties of feathers seemed to have no particular effect on him. Goose feathers, however, in his pillow invariably brought on an attack of asthma. On the other hand I have known people, who, if they used a hair pillow, were likely to sneeze during the night. It was not quite clear whether this was due to dust or to animal emanations in connection with the hair. Animal emanations in sensitive people can produce a very definite tendency to sneezing, though once their expectancy is aroused sneezing may be more easily evoked.

Yawning.—After coughing and sneezing, yawnis the next most interesting diaphragmatic movement. It is essentially a deep inspiration which increases the content of the thoracic cavity or chest very probably by one-half, for not only does the diaphragm descend to its fullest extent, but also the accessory muscles of respiration which lift the ribs and add to the content of the chest are brought into play. The action fills up the lungs with a large amount of fresh air and the complete expiration that follows drives out a large amount of residual air that has gradually been losing its vitalizing oxygen while remaining in the lungs. Undoubtedly yawning is due to an instinct, for it can be noticed even in very small children, in infants, long before the time when one would expect that any possible imitation of those near them could influence the child's action. It is, of course, shared by the animals, practically all of whom yawn at times. Probably nothing is more disturbing to the equanimity of the masters of dogs and, above all, the mistresses of cats than the calm way in which these animals will, in spite of human customs of politeness, yawn profoundly in the faces of their masters and mistresses. Animals yawn particularly on days when life has not been very active for them, and apparently the instinct is meant to make up to some extent for the deep breathing which comes naturally with exercise.

Human beings yawn when they are tired and sleepy and that is the physical reaction that yawning represents. When the tissues are tired we do not breathe very deeply and this is nature's way of getting more oxygen into the lungs and getting us ready for sleep and rest.

Yawning is however an index of mental tiredness as well as physical exhaustion. If a man has been sitting all day in a room doing one kind of monotonous work, in the late afternoon he is likely to do a good deal of yawning, and it may be rather hard for him to keep awake. He is not physically tired but he is mentally tired. Hearers who have to listen to a monotonous talker who has not very much to say are likely to yawn a great deal after a while. They may not be physically tired at all. If they were sitting at an interesting play there would not be a yawn for some two hours and a half. Mental tiredness is as effective as physical tiredness in producing yawning.

It is well known that yawning is very contagious, that is to say, if one person in a room yawns it will not be long before others will be doing the same thing. If an actor yawns on the stage some of the audience will begin to yawn before long, and it is perfectly possible to set most of a large audience yawning just as the result of yawning before them. They may not be tired, and this will happen just as well in the morning as it will in the afternoon or evening. There is something in us that tempts us to use our diaphragms in this way whenever we see others using theirs. Just why diaphragmatic movements are so contagious from a psychic standpoint is hard to say. The fact of its existence however must always be kept in mind whenever there is any question of trying to understand any of them. While yawning and laughing are separated as the opposite poles from each other, yet they have this one quality in common besides their being diaphragmatic activities, that they are both contagious. It has been suggested that it is much easier to control the contagiousness of yawning than of laughter, but, given certain circumstances, it is perfectly possible for people to be present where a great deal of laughter is being done without sharing it at all.

Hiccough.—A fourth form of physical diaphragmatic activity is represented by the hiccough.* The *Century Dictionary* describes it as "a quick, involuntary respiratory movement of the dia-

---

* In its present spelling the word hiccough serves to complete the variety of pronunciations of the syllable *ough* in English into the mystical number seven. In a book on laughter it may be noted that all seven of them are brought together in the single phrase—*though the rough cough and hiccough plough me thoroughly through.* It is no laughing matter, however, for the poor foreigner learning English to try to make his way clear through this maze of sound, all represented by a single combination of letters.

phragm, brought suddenly to a stop by an involuntary closing of the glottis," that is, the bringing together of the vocal cords in such a way as to shut off the intake of the breath. This produces the characteristic noise. The word is very interesting in its modern form, hiccough, because it has been modified to conform with the idea that the action is somehow related to cough, and therefore the word should be spelled so as to indicate that relationship. The original form of the word, hiccup, or as it was earlier written hickup or sometimes hickope, is imitative of the sound that occurs in connection with the action.

Hiccoughs are brought about by two sets of irritations. One of these is in the esophagus or swallowing tube in the neighborhood of the larynx that is at the upper end of the tube. The other is caused by irritation of the diaphragm. The first of these is the familiar hiccough that all of us have experienced. If we try to swallow something in a hurry, especially food that is rather dry, that has not been chewed very well, in the process of forcing it down the throat something happens that brings about hiccoughs. It is a warning that food is being passed to the stomach insufficiently prepared. This will usually be relieved by a series of swallows of water or some other fluid, especially either very warm or very cold fluid. If we fail to chew even the softer foods, such as potato or bread, and swallow them in rather large pieces, hiccoughs are likely to result. Apparently, there is some interference, in the swallowing process, with the larynx and its activities, and as that is the avenue for breath, which is so important, nature at once reacts to bring about a lessening of irritation, or even slight interference though it may be, with the larynx. Even water, if the attempt is made to force it down in large amounts when we are in a hurry, will sometimes bring on hiccoughs, so that there is evidently a very watchful sentinel on guard at this point to prevent any hampering of laryngeal activity.

The other mode of hiccoughs is due to direct irritation of the diaphragm, and is often a rather dangerous symptom. When peritonitis occurs, that, is inflammation of the inner lining of the abdominal cavity, if this spreads to the under side of the diaphragm, hiccoughs will result, in certain cases at least. Often it is extremely difficult to stop the hiccoughs, and all the ordinary remedies have no effect. Almost needless to say, peritonitis is an extremely dangerous affection and likely to be fatal. Hence the tradition that if a very sick person begins to hiccough, a fatal termination is likely to occur. Abscess of the liver has been known to cause hiccough, though probably the reason for it is the spread of some of the inflammation or inflammatory process to the peritoneal layer of the diaphragm in this region. Certain affections of the spleen are said to cause hiccough, and these are not so dangerous as the hiccough that is due to peritonitis, or to abscess of the liver.

The inflammatory condition acts directly on the diaphragm and causes it to make the involuntary spasmodic movements in imitation of the similar activity which occurs as the result of the reflex that is meant to protect the larynx from interference. The hiccough completes the list of physical activities in connection with the diaphragm, and while hiccough is said sometimes to be contagious, this is very rare. It may be purely psychoneurotic.

MENTAL DIAPHRAGM ACTIVITIES

These four, coughing, sneezing, yawning, and hiccoughing, are what may be called the physical diaphragm activities. Two, at least, of them have distinct mental factors that influence them, and sneezing and hiccough may occur under certain circumstances in a heightened mental state of expectancy. There are three other diaphragm activities, sighing, sobbing, and laughing, that are almost entirely dependent on mental states, though there are certain slight physical factors in their production. Tickling will produce laughter, sobbing and sighing are contagious when heard, and the visual image of sighing or sobbing will lead to imitation. All three of these convulsive diaphragmatic actions represent relief from pent up feelings. The consideration of sighing and sobbing in connection with laughter brings this out very well. To consider any one of these diaphragm activities without the others, is to lose sight of the background on which they must all be considered. Laughing can be much better understood as a perfectly natural process that has a definite meaning for body and mind, after the consideration of coughing, sneezing, yawning, sighing and sobbing, than could possibly be the case without due reflection on these cognate activities.

Sighing.—The least important of the diaphragm

activities is sighing. There is much more of it now than there used to be because we have so many more psychoneuroses than before. The psychoneurotics have a very definite tendency to pity themselves, and they express that by heaving "deep-sized" sighs. In the older time the sighing was mainly confined to young folks who were in love, and lovers' sighs were a favorite expression of the poets. Shakespeare said, "Love is a smoke raised with a fume of sighs." There was always something of self-pity in them. It is, of course, very well known that sighing also is contagious. If a young person in a room alone with another young person sighs it is very probable that another sigh will be heard before long. Even among neurotic people if they are thrown much together and they tell each other the stories of their ills and ails, the sighs they heave will be responded to by sighs on the part of others, and probably nothing is worse for such patients than the mutual reaction that thus occurs. Whenever my neurotic patients sigh deeply I always make it a point to sigh in return, but this is meant to show them what they are doing. Many a man or woman, and I think the men more than the women, who is sighing deeply every few minutes over himself and his ailment is not aware at all of the fact that he is doing it, and sometimes to imitate him is the best possible way to bring this fact into his consciousness.

Sighing has a very definite physical effect in producing a certain amount of depression of spirit. It is a sign of discouragement, but serves to emphasize it. It is a little bit like pulling the corners of the mouth down. It has been said that any one who deliberately turns the corners of his lips up, even though he has no feeling of smiling when he begins it will have a definite tendency to smile, and above all, have the feeling which accompanies it before long. On the other hand, if he pulls the corners of his lips down, he will have a rather definite tendency to feel glum and depressed. Almost the same thing is true with regard to sighing. It makes you feel that there is something that you would like to get that you cannot. It is an external manifestation of the fact that you feel that you are deserving of pity. Its contagiousness is not so marked as other diaphragmatic activities, but there is a definite element of that connected with the process.

Sobbing.—Perhaps the best understanding of sighing may be obtained from the fact that the definition of the word "sob" ordinarily given is that it is "a strong, convulsive sigh" (*Century*). A sob itself is defined as a convulsive heaving of the breast and inspiration of breath under the impulse of painful emotion, and accompanied by weeping. To sob is to weep with convulsive catchings of the breath. Ordinarily, a sigh is not considered to be related so closely to sobbing, but an analysis of it will show these definitions to be correct. Our contempt for sobbing, unless there is some very good reason for it, is demonstrated by our use of the word "sob-sisters" to designate feminine reporters who make it their business to get the stories of criminals and then retell them in such ways as will sentimentally touch the heart of the public and make them feel pity for the criminals, though our pity should be reserved more particularly for the victims of the criminals.

Sobbing is another of these convulsive movements of the diaphragm, however, that is distinctly contagious. Wandering evangelists, who depend for their success on the touching of people so as to make them express their religious feelings in public, know very well that if one or two people can be gotten to sob over their sins, or their relations with the Almighty, others will surely follow, and such activities are distinctly contagious. At a funeral, if some relative who has not been present before, comes from a distance and sets up a sobbing, others in the room will almost surely follow. Some of this of course is merely conventional, and is due to the fact that people think that under these circumstances they should make some public manifestation of their grief, but not a little of it is due to that tendency to contagion which exists in practically all the diaphragmatic activities.

The effect may be produced entirely through the mind, and without any reality of affection or sense of loss. Sobbing is sometimes heard in the theater in connection with a very pathetic play, and there are various catches of the breath between a sigh and a sob that may be noticed under these circumstances. The sobbing is practically always accompanied by moisture in the eyes, though it may not be accompanied by true weeping. All the diaphragm activities, however, are associated with hypersecretion of tears and their appearance on the lashes, or even down the cheeks. In coughing, tears run, but so do they also in yawning, and of course they are present in sneezing, and, curiously enough, laughing is practically always accompanied by the presence of tears in the eyes. It would seem as though there were some reflex connection between movements of the diaphragm, beyond those for respiration, and the flow of tears.

Laughing.—Finally there remains laughter as a diaphragmatic activity for which there seems to be less purpose than for any of the others mentioned. It is, of course, the contrary of sighing or sobbing, and these three are quite different from coughing, yawning and sneezing, which are almost entirely physical reflexes, though, as we have seen, there are mental elements in them, and above all they are contagious. Sighing, sobbing and laughing are dependent almost entirely on mental states, though of course a laugh may be almost a purely physical reflex. Laughing can be produced by tickling, that is by touching the fingers lightly especially over the parts of the body that are nearest to the diaphragm, though of course the soles of the feet and, to a certain extent, the palm of the hand are ticklish. Ticklishness has been the subject of a good deal of conjecture. Tickling brings about at once a squirming movement or a wriggle that tends to get the part tickled away from the touches. It is extremely important that the soles of the feet should be protected from injury, for a man's life may depend on his ability to get away from danger, and he cannot do so with rapidity if his feet are sore. The other ticklish portions of the body are in intimate relations with our most important organs, so that the wriggle away from the touch is easy to understand as a protective reflex.

Just why this wriggle should be accompanied by a laugh, however, it has been difficult to understand. Very early in life, even before the end of the third month, if the fingers are passed lightly along the sides of the chest wall of infants, especially down near the diaphragm, they will wriggle and laugh. Tickling in older folks is usually not pleasant, but children manifestly like it. They respond very much in the same way as a dog does to rubbing. They will wriggle and laugh and turn themselves over on their backs in order to allow the tickling to continue. Light touches of the soles of the feet seem to have the same effect on children, and cause them to laugh, but in grown folk touches of the soles of the feet become very unpleasant, and it is sometimes said that one of the most awful modes of torture is to put a man to death by tickling the soles of his feet. Savage tribes know this and have occasionally used it as special torture for traitors or the murderers of chiefs.

Laughing is, however, mainly a response to mental stimuli, and this is true above all in adults. Just why we laugh as the result of hearing jokes or seeing something that excites our risibilities, that is, why the risibilities are excited, we do not know. We have had many explanations, but most of them contradict each other, and the more you read of them the more you realize how little is understood about the subject. For instance, Bergson says that "emotion is a foe to laughter." He suggests that "the comic demands something like a momentary anesthesia of the heart," that is, of that faculty in which are our kindly feelings. He adds, "The appeal of the comic is to the intelligence pure and simple." On the other hand, Herbert Spencer says, "Strong feeling, mental or physical, is the general cause of laughter." Of course it is possible to reconcile the two views by making due allowances for the way in which the two men use the words, and yet, even then, these two authorities will be poles apart in what they consider to be the element that makes people laugh. MacDougall suggests that laughter is an instinct and therefore, as it were, connected with our bodily state rather than with our mind, though most writers on the subject have emphasized the mental condition.

What we are interested in here is the fact that laughter represents probably the most important of these diaphragm activities, all of which have a definite purpose for the safeguarding of health and the prevention of disease development. When we are young laughter is almost entirely instinctive, and we laugh at almost nothing so that it is very evident that nature intended that this function should be exercised without the necessity for much provocation. Nature is as provident in this as with regard to other instincts. From our youngest years we know when we need to take food, and when we have enough, and without these precious instincts the matter of raising us would be very difficult indeed. Laughter was meant to continue throughout life, and does for a great many people, but there are others who fail to realize its value and pervert their instinct. There are people who do the same thing with regard to eating. They eat either too much or too little, and it is surprising how many of them who complain of distress are just not giving their stomachs enough to do. A good many grown-ups who fail to laugh as much as they should are disturbing another precious instinct in the same way.*

---

* The diaphragm has more than a little to do with various disturbing activities of the stomach. The belching of gas, for instance, is often thought to be merely mechanical, in the sense of representing the eructation of gaseous material whenever the stomach gets overdistended with it, until there is a sort of forcing of the cardiac orifice of the stomach into which the esophagus leads. It is now recognized, however, that the diaphragm has much to do with this and that when the pressure on the stomach goes beyond a certain point, it is a downward movement of the diaphragm that causes the air to be expelled.

In something the same way there are patients who have a definite tendency to swallow air. There is a nice long Greek name for them, the aërophages or air eaters. This swallowed air may become quite uncomfortable, and not a few of these patients feel that they are sufferers from indigestion or from gastro-intestinal disturbance because they have gaseous distention of the stomach and intestines. The gaspiness which causes the swallowing of air is diaphragmatic in origin and represents something of a cross between a sigh and a yawn. Some people get the habit of it, and it is a source of considerable annoyance at times when they are nervous.

There is another manifestation connected with the stomach, somewhat nervous in character, but associated with a special diaphragm activity. This is what is known as rumination, or, to use the Greek term, merycism, which is applied only to human beings. It is the raising of food and chewing it again, and then swallowing it. The animals known as the ruminants, that is, the chewers of their cud, do this regularly, and man does it occasionally. Usually those who do it are rather nervous individuals, and sometimes they have mental trouble of one kind or another.

Certain forms of vomiting are associated not so much with nausea as with movements of the diaphragm, especially of spasmodic character. This is well known to occur in connection with certain tumors of the brain that have for a very characteristic symptom expulsive vomiting. This comes on very suddenly, without any preliminary nausea, and the contents of the stomach may be ejected to a distance. This is much more like a cough than a real vomiting action.

Vomiting in connection with seasickness is nearly always diaphragmatic in character rather than due to stomach disturbance. The origin of the trouble is to be found in the organ of equilibrium. When this is disturbed, as happens by the up and down movement of a vessel, vomiting occurs because of a spasmodic movement of the diaphragm. This does not always cause the upsetting of the stomach immediately, but its movements lead to a reversed action of the intestines, and the pouring into the stomach of intestinal secretion which proves intensely nauseating. The diaphragm has more to do with it than the stomach itself, very probably, though of course the initiative comes from the semicircular canals in the organ of equilibrium. Children learn that they can make themselves dizzy by going round and round, and sometimes they play a game at that, but suffer from vomiting as a consequence if it is continued beyond a certain limit.

Physicians who see much of seasickness, as for instance ship doctors, know that a great many people make their own seasickness by thinking about it. Even though they have taken no food and only a little fluid, they proceed to vomit, but the intermediary for the activity is the diaphragm. In a word, this big muscle to which the Greeks attributed the highest function in the body, thought, has a great deal more to do with influencing various functions in the body than is usually supposed.

INDEX